DECODING KOREAN ACUPUNCTURE

Korean Constitutional Acupuncture, Joseon
Acupuncture, & Sa Ahm Acupuncture

ISBN: 9798790929939

Cover design by: Art Painter
Library of Congress Control Number: 2018675309
Printed in the United States of America

CONTENTS

DECODING KOREAN ACUPUNCTURE

- Korean Constitutional Acupuncture,
Joseon Acupuncture,
& Sa Ahm acupuncture -

ANGIE YOUNG KIM PH.D.

TABLE OF CONTENTS

Chapter 3 Sa Ahm acupuncture

Introduction

Basic Theories

Hand Yangming Large Intestine Meridian

1. Indications
2. Case studies

Foot Yangming Large Stomach Meridian

1. Indications
2. Case studies

Hand Taiyin Lung Meridian

1. Indications
2. Case studies

Foot Taiyin Spleen Meridian

1. Indications
2. Case studies

Hand Tai Yang Small Intestine Meridian

1. Indications
2. Case studies

Foot Tai Yang Urinary Bladder Meridian

1. Indications
2. Case studies

Hand Shao Yin Heart Meridian

1. Indications
2. Case studies

Foot Shao Yin Kidney Meridian

1. Indications
2. Case studies

Hand Shao Yang San Jiao Meridian

1. Indications
2. Case studies

Foot Shao Yang Gall Bladder Meridian

1. Indications
2. Case studies

Hand Jueyin Pericardium meridian

1. Indications
2. Case studies

Foot Jueyin Liver meridian

1. Indications
2. Case studies

Chapter 4 Conculsion

Appendix

Bibliography

Acknowledgement

FOREWORD

I am so excited to reveal the three most clinically effective methods of Korean acupuncture since it has been working successfully in my seventeen years of acupuncture practice as a form of Traditional Asian Medicine.

Studying Traditional Asian Medicine is like the blind men touching a giant elephant to learn what it is like. With thousands years of history, there is a myriad of literature and theories, and not only is it hard to perceive the big picture, it takes effort to distinguish between the gems and pebbles.

As a practitioner, it is also very easy to be stuck in one outstanding theory and delude oneself that he or she has mastered the whole Traditional Asian Medicine. However, Traditional Asian Medicine itself is a masterpiece that has not been completed.

Here are three pieces of a picture of the giant elephant of Traditional Acupuncture that have been practiced in Korea but not fully adopted in traditional Asian medical education in the US. The first is Korean Constitutional Medicine that is developed by Dr. Lee Jema and Dr. Kwon Dowon, the second is Joseon Acupuncture technique that is based on 'The Empirical fomulas of Acupuncuture' of Dr. Heo Im, and the third is Sa Ahm acupuncture that is also known as four needle technique.

These three can be indicators in the clinical practice of acupuncture. I believe these are crucial clues to putting all the pieces together in acupuncture practice, yet need to be further studied and proved in clinical settings.

In the section of Joseon acupuncture, the authentic deep needling technique is introduced that is developed a few hundred years ago and used thicker and longer needles. However, it is recommended to start from a conservative approach with needles of smaller diameter at first and with shorter retaining time. After you practice on numerous patients, you will eventually know which guage of needles are needed to use for which patients.

I hope this book can provide acupuncturists with stepping stones on the journey to mastering Korean style acupuncture, which will lead to excellence in their practice.

Angie Young Kim, Ph.D., L.Ac.

ABOUT THE AUTHOR

Angie Young Kim

Angie Kim has practiced acupuncture and traditional Asian herbal medicine successfully in California since 2005. Her vision is to contribute herself to the development of traditional Asian Medicine by healing people in the most natural way and sharing her knowledge and experience with others.

Angie holds a doctorate in Traditional Asian Medicine. On graduating Summa Cum Laude from Emperor's College of Traditional Oriental Medicine, she has taken her continuing trainings including Korean Medicine Program at Kyung Hee University of South Korea, Korean Sasang Constitutional Medicine Program with Dr. Man Hur who is the third generation Sasang Medicine practitioner, and studies of Korean style acupuncture with great Korean Medicine scholars.

She also lectured at Dongguk University in Los Angeles, California, and School of Alternative Medicine, Life University in Gardena, California. Now her passion is to share her clinical experience of Korean Constitutional Medicine and acupuncture with peer acupuncturists and herbalists all over the world.

CHAPTER 1

KOREAN CONSTITUTIONAL ACUPUNCTURE

Korean Constitutional Medicine originated from the philosophy of Sasang Constitutional Medicine(SCM), which was developed by Dr. Jema Lee, in his book <Dongui Suse Bowon(東醫壽世保元)> in 1894. Sasang(四象) means 'Four shapes' or 'Four Images', which shows that one of the basic ideas of Dr. Lee is 'internal energy, external shape (氣裏形表)[1]', meaning internal energy is manifested externally. Based on this concept, four different body types were identified. Those are Tai Yang(Greater Yang), Shao Yang(Lesser Yang), Tai Yin(Greater Yin), and Shao Yin(Lesser Yin).

As Dr. Lee wrote in his book, the division of these 4 constitutions originated from the Nei Jing. However, it has to be pointed out that his creative thinking about the division into four constitutions is due to the relative functional size of the organs, which is a remarkable idea in the history of Eastern Medicine.[2] This is also the first approach based on the Yin and Yang theory that focused on individual difference rather than the difference of the pathological symptoms.

Although these 4 terms of Tai Yang, Tai Yin, Shao Yang, and Shao Yin may sound familiar, since they are also used in the 6 channel theory of Shang Han Lun[3], the actual concepts are completely different in that Shang Han Lun described them as the stages of disease progression not as body types.

Dr. Song Il-Byung, a Traditional Eastern Medicine doctor and professor in Kyung Hee university in Korea reinterpreted the Sasang philosophy in comparison with the one in Nei Jing, stating;

"The philosophy of the Nei Jing is based on the belief that everything is classified into Five primary substances (wood, fire, earth, metal, water). Compared with the Nei Jing, the philosophy of Sasang medicine believes that 'Things exist, Principles exist' and 'Human mind, Human body' on top of a system that groups things into four images. Through this introduction of a new philosophy, Sasang medicine could set up four constitutions, each with its own body-shape and physiology and pathology of the internal organs."[4]

In the article *Sasang Constitutional Medicine as a Holistic Tailored Medicine*, Dr. Lee's unique idea of the 4 constitutional organ system is well described.

"An explanation of internal visceral systems, SCM uses the same terminology found in TCM (Traditional Chinese Medicine), but each creates a different system of classification. SCM regards the heart as the king among the five viscera, which is equivalent to the mind. Departing from the visceral theory in TCM, where viscera are assigned in pairs, zang and fu, SCM assumes a theory of visceral groups: the lung, kidney, liver and spleen groups. The lung group includes the lungs, tongue, esophagus region, ears, brain and skin. The spleen group consists of the spleen, stomach, breasts, eyes and tendons. The constituents of the liver group are the liver, small intestine, nose, lumbar region and muscles. The kidney group has the kidney, large intestine, urethra, bladder, mouth and bones. Among these groups, it is believed that specific inter-regulatory relations are present between specific pairs of visceral group. As such, visceral groups are classified into two pairs: one consists of the spleen and the kidney group and the other is composed of the lung and the liver group. The relation in each pair of visceral groups is akin to the balancing state of a seesaw. In this respect, a hyperactive state in one group leads to a relatively deficient state in its counterpart. The state of hyperactivity in the lung group leads to a hypoactive state of the liver in Tai Yang types, but vice versa in Tai Yin types. Finally, the state of hyperactivity in the spleen group leads to a hypoactive state of the kidney group in Shao Yang types, but vice versa in Shao Yin types."[5]

Based on the imbalances defined by these inter-regulatory relations, each body type manifests uniquely in terms of appearance, physical traits, mental and emotional characteristics, physiological and pathological signs and symptoms, etc.

Dr. Song, in his book *Sasang Medicine Made Easy*, suggested that constitutional diagnosis should be made comprehensively based on all three of the appearances, the nature of the disposition, and the pathological symptoms. Especially, in the earlier practice of Sasang constitutional medicine, hasty conclusions considering only one or two of these aspects can lead to a wrong diagnosis.

It is well known among Eastern Herbalists that the right formula determined from the right diagnosis can make a great improvement in a patient's condition but the other way around can not only accomplish nothing but may even make the patient worse. Especially, in Sasang constitutional medical practice, the right formula used for the right person is the key to treat any condition. Although Sasang Constitutional Medicine may not be a perfect system for treating people, it can provide us with main indicators that lead us in the right direction. When herbal practitioners can grasp the idea of grouping the 4 constitutions, they will come a step closer to being able to use not only Sasang constitutional formulas but also any other formulas including Shang Han Lun formulas.

With herbal prescription as the main treatment method of Sasang constitutional Medicine, Dr. Lee Je-Ma thought highly of Dr. Zhang Zhongjing, and quoted many symptom presentations and formulas from Dr. Zhang's Shang Han Lun. However, he described them according to his system of Sasang constitutional theory, not following the 6 Channel theory of Shang Han Lun. He also created his own formulas that he deemed beneficial for each constitution.

The details of herbal formula practices in SCM are explained in my other book, <New paradigms for Shang Han Lun>. This book is mainly focused on how this concept of SCM is developed in acupuncture practice along with other powerful Korean traditional acupuncture techniques.

Four body type differentiation

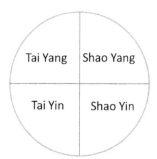

Tai Yang type : Excess Lung with Deficient Liver
Tai Yin type : Excess Liver with Deficient Lung
Shao Yang type : Excess Spleen with Deficient Kidney
Shao Yin type : Excess Kidney with Deficinet Spleen

<Four burner theory related to body trunk portion>

Upper burner:	The portion that Lung governs (Lung, Trachea and Esophagus-Expectorate and breathing out function
Upper mid burner:	The Portion that Spleen governs (Spleen and Stomach)- Receiving food
Lower mid burner:	The Portion that Liver governs (Liver and Small Intestine) -processing food
Lower burner:	The Portions that Kidney governs (Kidney and Large intestine) -Elimination

< Standard facial features of the sasang constitution>

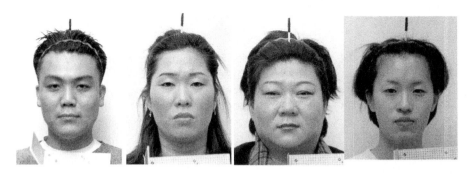

In 2012, the department of Sasang Constitutional Medicine of Kyunghee University Oriental Medical Center released a report after researching on Sasang Constitution Diagnosis using facial features. The related pictures of 4 constitutions that the research provided are available online. The pictures above shows more prominent features of each body type, which is presented by Dr. Hong seok chul. The first picture is the face of Tai Yang body type, the second is Shao Yang, the third is Tai Yin, and the last one is Shao Yin.

However, this is only one aspect of constitutional diagnosis. As Dr. Song suggested in his book , constitutional diagnosis should be made comprehensively based on all three of the appearances, the nature of the disposition, and the pathological symptoms.

1.   Shao Yin Constitution

Shaoyins usually have a well-developed hip area and a less developed chest area. The lower body is more developed than the upper. The skin tends to be soft and relatively moist. Muscle tone cannot be developed easily for this body type thus generally weak muscles or even sagging muscles in seniors can be found. They tend to hunch forward due to their weak chest area. For the face, the lower jaw is relatively bigger and well developed.

It is said that Shaoyins tend to be petite and have a small physique, but in the US with its variety of ethnic group, there are a variety of Shao Yin body types, some tall and slim, and some are even corpulent. In my clinical experience, Shaoyins in US are mostly taller than Shaoyangs. The statue of Venus shows the classic female appearance of a Shao Yin body type, with a smooth body line and soft skin. The feet of this type are usually very cold to the touch due to strong Kidney water energy. People with the Shao Yin body type usually complain of low energy due to weaker Spleen energy, and generally experience an aversion to cold and less perspiration.

Shaoyins have a tendency to introversion and a feminine nature, and are docile, self-possessed, and circumspect. They would rather stay at home than go out, and are always nervous that things might be wrong, even with little things. They are usually detailed oriented and very organized, so they can accomplish goals when they are determined and push ahead with a given project. However, due to their passive attitude and low energy, it is easy for them to get complacent and idle, not being able to overcome obstacles.

All the above physical and mental traits are manifestations originating from organ imbalances of the large kidneys and the small Spleen in Shao Yin body types. The size of organs referred to in SCM original texts means the energetic and functional dimension of the organs, not the actual size of the organs.

People with Shao Yin body types, due to Spleen weakness, tend to have digestive problems when they are not in good condition, so it is said that Shaoyins are healthy when they digest well. And most of their symptoms get worse when attacked by cold pathogens due to strong kidney water energy. Therefore, it is said that the pathological symptoms of the Shao Yin body type are mainly characterized by symptoms caused by the Stomach Cold and the Spleen/Kidney Yang Deficiency, which are poor digestion, incessant diarrhea, and streaming sweat, etc.

2.   Shao Yang Constitution

Points of differentiation

Shaoyangs have a well-developed chest area which corresponds to the Spleen, but their hip area, which corresponds to the Kidneys, is relatively smaller and weaker. Some Shaoyang women with narrower hips may experience difficulty in conceiving due to weaker Kidney energy. Their face is usually smaller and oval with a thin and pointy jaw. Their eyes radiate a sharp and intense look. They tend to be outspoken and move quickly and do things in a hasty manner, which makes them look careless. Among celebrities, Bruce Lee has most physical traits of a typical Shao Yang constitution. Some Shaoyangs, especially in their later life, still can gain weight, but most Shaoyangs exude swift and agile impression. I better avoid mentioning too many celebrity names because physical aspects are not the only factor differentiating body types, but are only one of many, including psychological and pathophysiological aspects.

Shaoyangs are active, animated, and cheerful, and also good at exploring new experiences and pushing ahead with plans. However, they tend to be impatient in sticking to one project, and end up not being able to finish. They also love to take care of other's business rather than their own due to their tendency to extraversion. This can arouse anxiety and fearfulness, causing problems in family relationships, and if this goes to the extreme and they totally pursue achievements in the outside world, they can get more anxious and impulsive and do things on a whim without mature consideration.

Shaoyangs have a strong Spleen but weak kidneys. Therefore, their digestive systems are relatively strong, but their reproductive systems can be on the weaker side. It is said that Shaoyangs are healthy and sound if their bowel movements are regular. When they get constipated, they become vulnerable to pathogenic factors. Only 2-3 days of constipation still can cause Shaoyangs heaviness and stuffiness in their chest, which can lead to other serious illness. The congested feeling in the chest implies stagnation of excess yang (fire/heat) due to Kidney Yin (water/cold) deficiency. Prolonged imbalance of excess Yang and deficient Yin in Shao Yang constitution can later manifest as various types of Warm Febrile Diseases.

3.   Tai Yin Constitution

Taiyins have strong Liver and weak Lungs. The Liver's function is to store blood and the Liver Qi is easily stagnated. Thus Taiyins naturally accumulate Qi and blood easily rather than eliminating it, which causes them to gain weight especially around the waist area that corresponds to the Liver. Their face is usually round or square, their skin is relatively thick, and they usually sweat easily. The famous actress Conchata Ferrell, who played Berta the housekeeper for the sitcom *Two and a Half Men*, is a classic example of Tai Yin body type.

As for personality, Taiyins are mostly calm, laidback, patient, persistent, and pragmatic. They have a great sense of responsibility, and eventually accomplish their goals. They tend to prefer staying still and are unwilling to move around. This causes them to only take care of their own business and family and not consider the outside world. If this goes to the extreme, it can arouse fear in their mind and they can become more mistrustful, closed minded, and cowardly. As their organ imbalance causes a natural accumulation of substances rather than an elimination, when it comes to the imbalance of their life, they can become greedy and possessive, not sharing anything but constantly trying to acquire more.

Their physical condition is good when they sweat freely. If there is no sweat with firmer skin and closed pores, it indicates an unhealthy state for Taiyins and can lead to a more serious illness. The accumulated waste in their body can be somewhat released with sweating during exercise. While Shaoyins get tired after sweating, Taiyins become refreshed and revitalized after sweating.

The overaccumulation of substances combined with the slow metabolism in Taiyin can cause heat congestion that leads to Dryness in the Lungs and Heat in the Liver. More often than not Taiyin can get constipated easily due to a high appetite and slow metabolism. However, diarrhea or dysentery in this constitution can be counted as a more serious condition. Overall, we can say that Taiyins are healthy when they are able to release their accumulated substances through sweat, urination and bowel movement. The malfunction of these three such as no sweating, urinary difficulty and constipation can generate Dry Heat Syndrome, which is the main characteristic of the pathological syndrome of Tai Yin body type.

4.   Tai Yang Constitution

Tai Yang constitution, known as the greater Yang compared to the lesser Yang (Shao Yang), has more noticeable development in upper body (yang) and a less developed lower body (yin). Therefore, their Pectoralis Major is well developed, and the head and neck area is also bigger than on other body types. The lower portion from the waist down, which corresponds to the Liver, is rather weak. Their standing posture looks unstable due to their small buttocks and weak legs. Their facial characteristics are clearly defined and rugged with sharp and piercing eyes creating an intense and aggressive look. Taiyangs are the rarest body type: imagine the character Hercules in the Walt Disney animated film.

Taiyangs make friends easily because they are very social and have good communication skills. They are extremely creative, highly intelligent and naturally inquisitive. Due to their excessive Yang energy, they always want to move forward and are typically hotheaded and reckless. Yang is masculine energy, and when this energy goes to the extreme, Taiyangs can be cocky, self-indulgent, self-righteous, and easily fall into heroism.

Taiyangs possess strong lungs and a weak liver. As opposed to Taiyins, they naturally disperse Qi and eliminate substances easily rather than accumulating them. Therefore, most of their issues stem from too much dispersal of Yang energy upward and too little storage of body substances. Taiyangs are healthy if they urinate well, because urination indicates that the energy is moving downward within the body. If their energy goes upward too much, it can cause excessive foamy saliva, dysphagia, and vomiting, which needs to be addressed immediately. Excess in the upper body leads to deficiency in the lower body. The associated symptoms are lower back pain, weakness in the lower body, and difficulty walking. If symptoms get more serious, they may also experience weight loss and severe fatigue, not even wanting to talk or move.

Eight body type differentiation

There have been efforts to develop SCM from the overall approach of evidence based medicine (EBM), integrating both western allopathic and holistic traditional medicine. The studies vary from investigations into diagnostic methods to improve accuracy of diagnosis to explorations of the development of systems of constitution.

Among those, Eight Constitutional Medicine(ECM) by Dr. Kwon Dowon is the most creative outcome in that he revealed the strengths and weaknesses of all ten organs along with the activity of sympathetic and parasympathetic nerve systems in each of the eight different body types and applied his theory to acupuncture treatments.

"The human body consists of 10 organs altogether: five solid organs and five hollow organs. From the point of conception, these organs develop and fall into an order of strong and weak, and the groupings of these orders that are distinguishable from each other total eight. This is the fundamental, underlying principle of the eight constitutions, with the strengths and weakness of the organs being directly related to their size.

That said, the condition in which the liver is the largest organ with the nine remaining organs ordered according to strength and weakness is called Hepatonia, while the condition where the pancreas is largest is called Pancretonia, that with the stomach is the largest Gastrotonia, that with the lungs as the largest Pulmotonia, that with the colon as the largest Colonotonia, that with the kidneys as largest Renotonia, and that with the bladder as the largest Vesicotonia.

Among these eight constitutions, there are four in which the sympathetic nervous system is always in a tense state. The grouping of these is called sympathicotonia, and includes Pulmotonia, Colonotonia, Renotonia, and Vesicotonia. The other grouping is called Vagotonia, in which the parasympathetic nervous system is always in a tense state, and includes Hepatonia, Cholecystonia, Pancreotonia, and Gastrotonia. One of the characteristics of those with a constitution grouped under

Vagotonia is that beneficial for them drink caffeinated coffee or other caffeinated drinks. Those who fall under the category of Sympathicotonia should not drink caffeinated coffee.

Recently, the results of a comparative examination of the degree of activity of Amylase in the saliva of people from each of eight constitutions at Dong-A University in Busan (South Korea) revealed that Amylase was high in the four Sympathicotonia constitutions, while it was low in the four Vagotonia constitution."

From *Eight Constitutional Medicine: An overview* by Dr. Kuon Dowon

Based on the ECM theory, the eight constitutions are as follow.

- Renotonia (water yang): Kidney > Lung > Liver >Heart > Pancreas
- Vesicotonia(water yin): Urinary Bladder > Gall Bladder > Small Intestine > Large Intestine> Stomach
- Hepatonia (wood yang): Liver > Kidney > Heart > Pancreas > Lung
- Cholecystonia (wood yin): Gall Bladder > Small Intestine >Stomach> Urinary Bladder > Large Intestine
- Pulmotonia (metal yang): Lung > Pancreas > Heart > Kidney > Liver
- Colonotonia(metal yin): Large Intestine>Urinary Bladder>Stomach>Small Intestine> Gall Bladder
- Pancreotonia (earth yang): Pancreas > Heart > Liver > Lung > Kidney
- Gastrotonia (earth yin): Stomach > Large Intestine >Small Intestine > Gall Bladder > Urinary Bladder

- From *heavenly regimen* by CMC research group (Korean version)

In ECM, the administration of vitamin supplements and medications per each body type has been studied in addition to food regimens. For example, vitamin B supplement is the most beneficial for Shaoyins, vitamin E supplement is for Shaoyangs, and vitamin D supplement for Taiyins. And taking a tablet of baby Aspirin everyday can prevent many diseases in the body type of Hepatonia.

Further studies are needed on the efficacy of western medicines in relation to each body type. Due to Americans' higher use of western medical drugs, this study would also play a role in discerning body types as a diagnostic method.

Dr. Kwon's main achievement is that he invented 8 body type acupuncture along with food regimens, whereas Dr. Lee Jema mostly focused on herbal formulas according to his 4 constitutional theory.

However, Dr. Kwon's main diagnostic method to differentiate the 8 constitutions, which is the pulse diagnosis, is quite hard to grasp for most acupuncturists due to its extremely subjective nature of approach. That is why numerous Korean medicine doctors have been trying to develop more tangible diagnostic methods utilizing traditional 4 constitutional medicine theory, even if Dr. Kuon insists that each constitution in his ECM theory exists independently not belonging to any of 4 constitutions of Dr. Lee.

This book introduces Korean eight constitutional acupuncture following the diagnostic methods of Sasang constitutional medicine that are developed further in a modern way. Therefore, the eight constitutions from this perspective are divided into eight from the 4 constitutions as below.

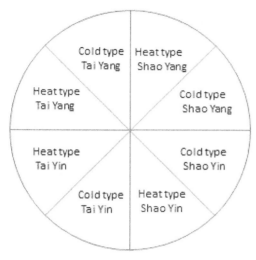

* Heat type Tai Yang Constitution
  : Tai Yang type with Shao Yang quality
* Cold type Tai Yang Constitution
  : Tai Yang type with Shao Yin quality
* Heat type Shao Yang Constitution
  : Shao Yang type with Tai Yang quality
* Cold type Shao Yang Constitution
  : Shao Yang type with Tai Yin quality
* Heat type Tai Yin Constitution
  : Tai Yin type with Shao Yang quality
* Cold type Tai Yin Constitution
  : Tai Yin type with Shao Yin quality
* Heat type Shao Yin Constitution
  : Shao Yin type with Tai Yang quality
* Cold type Shao Yin Constitution
  : Shao Yin type with Tai Yin quality

In Sasang constitutional medicine, heat and cold is relative concept of subjective feeling or objective observation. Shaoyangs have the most heat, so can be called heat constitution. Taiyangs are the next, so can be called warm constitution. Taiyins are cool constitution, and Shaoyins are cold constitution. That being said, the normal temperature for all the constitution has a wide range from 97°F to 99°F.

In Korean Constitutional Acupuncture (KCA) as in the picture above, each body type is further divided into heat and cold type. This is based on observation that each constitution has two clearly different groups that have different physiological and pathological phenomena. It led to the different approach of treatments for 8 constitutions in terms of acupuncture and herbal formulas.

Although this KCA model followed Sasang constitutional diagnostic system that is further developed by modern contemporary Korean acupuncturists, the Zang Fu relation followed Traditional Chinese Medicine (TCM) theory, not following SCM. In the acupuncture clinical practice, this model is approved working for patients regardless of their ethnicity. Since Dr. Lee Jema never mentioned acupuncture with SCM but only explained herbal formulas in his book <Dongui Suse Bowon>, SCM formula practice is recommended to follow his own Zang Fu theory as described in my other book <New paradigms for Shang Han Lun>.

Dr. Lee's book <Dongui Suse Bowon> also provided the clue that the Sasang constitution could be further divided into eight as described in the table below.

	Exterior pattern	Interior pattern
Shao Yin	Kidney Heat-based Exterior Heat disease (→ Heat Shao Yin constitution)	Stomach Heat-based Interior Cold disease (→ Cold Shao Yin constitution)
Shao Yang	Spleen Cold-based Exterior Cold disease (→ Cold Shao Yang constitution)	Stomach Heat-based Interior Heat disease (→ Heat Shao Yang constitution)
Tai Yin	Epigastric Cold-based Exterior Cold disease (→ Cold Tai Yin constitution)	Liver Heat-based interior heat disease (→ Heat Tai Yin constitution)
Tai Yang	Exterior Origin Lower Back disease (→ Heat Tai Yang constitution)	Interior Origin Small Intestine disease (→ Cold Tai Yang constitution)

1. Heat Shao Yin Constitution (Shao Yin type with Tai Yang quality)

Kidney > Lung > Liver >Heart > Spleen

Urinary Bladder > Large Intestine > Gall Bladder > Small Intestine > Stomach

AKA. Water Yang body type. Renotonia.

Heat Shaoyins have the strongest Kidney and UB energy. The second strongest are the Lung and Large intestine. Their Liver and Gall bladder are relatively weaker, and their Spleen and Stomach are the weakest.

They usually have a well-developed hip area and shoulder area. Most of Heat Shaoyins are slim with long and slender legs. Even when they gain weight in some cases, the body is still relatively well proportioned.

Every actor who has played Superman and every actress who has played Wonder Woman most likely belongs to this body type.

According to Dr. Kwon, those of Renotonia are very thorough and scrupulous, preferring precision, harboring doubts, and not easily believing others without experiencing things for themselves. Such a constitution has difficulty in believing in the existence of God or gods. They are, however, also talented in work that organizes various facts of things.

Disease unique to those of this body type include sunstroke and habitual constipation while otherwise healthy.

- Beneficial food

Sweet / Brown rice, Chicken and Poultry, Lamb, Beef, Seaweeds, Cinnamon, Ginger, Green onion, Mustard, Red and black pepper, Sesame oil, Potato, Apple, Mango, Orange/Citrus, Tomato, Ginseng, Honey, Dates, Vitamin B group.

2. Cold Shao Yin Constitution (Shao Yin type with Tai Yin quality)

Kidney > Liver > Heart > Lung > Spleen

Urinary Bladder > Gall Bladder > Small Intestine > Large Intestine> Stomach

Also known as Water Yin body type. Vesicotonia.

Cold Shaoyins have the strongest Kidney and UB energy. The next strongest are the Liver and Gall bladder. Their Lung and Large intestine are relatively weaker, and their Spleen and Stomach are the weakest.

They usually have a well-developed hip area and a less developed chest area. Since their Lung energy is on the weaker side, the shoulder area is less developed as well. Most of Cold Shaoyins are thin and slim with less developed muscles. Especially their upper body is much less developed than other constitutions.

Dr. Kwon considered that those of Vesicotonia who are healthy tend to be small eaters. Although this appears attributable to the fact that they are either born with small stomachs or have no interest in eating, this is rather be the most ideal method of maintaining health for people of this constitution.

Disease unique to those of this body type are gastroptosis and lymphocytic leukemia.

• Beneficial food

Sweet / Brown rice, Potato, Corn, Sesame oil, Seaweeds, Chicken and Poultry, Lamb, Red and black pepper, Mustard, Cinnamon, Curry, Green onion, Ginger, Apple, Orange/Citrus, Tomato, Mango, Ginseng, Dates, Honey, Vitamin B group

3. Heat Shao Yang Constitution (Shao Yang type with Tai Yang quality)

Spleen > Lung > Liver >Heart > Kidney

Stomach > Large Intestine >Small Intestine > Gall Bladder > Urinary Bladder

AKA. Earth Yin Body type. Gastrotonia.

Heat Shaoyangs have the strongest Spleen and Stomach energy. The next strongest are the Lung and Large intestine. Their Liver and Gall bladder is relatively weaker, and their Kidney and Urinary Bladder are the weakest.

They usually have a well-developed chest area and a less developed hip area. Their muscles are also well developed. Due to their strong Lung energy, the voice is usually resonant and they like to talk. They can easily have frequent urination from an early age due to the weakest water energy.

Dr. Kwon regarded this Gastrotonia as a very rare constitution.

- Beneficial food

Barley, Rice, Red beans, Mung beans, Cucumber, Green Vegetables, All kinds of ocean fishes and shellfishes, Swellfish, Pork, Beef, Persimmon, Melons, Pineapple, Grapes, Strawberry, Banana, Aloe vera, Ice, Chocolate, Vitamin E.

4. Cold Shao Yang Constitution (Shao Yang type with Tai Yin quality)

Spleen > Heart > Liver > Lung > Kidney

Stomach > Small Intestine > Gall Bladder > Large Intestine> Urinary Bladder

AKA. Earth Yang body type. Pancreotonia.

Cold Shaoyangs have the strongest Spleen and Stomach energy. Their Liver and Gall bladder is relatively on the stronger side. The energy of Lung and Large Intestine is on the weaker side, and their Kidney and Urinary Bladder are the weakest.

They usually have a well-developed chest area and a less developed hip area. Their muscles are also well developed. They can easily have low back pain due to the deficiency of Kidney energy.

Since their Wood energy is on the stronger side, they still can gain weight easily. However, they still don't gain as much as Tai Yin type, because of the active and outgoing nature of dominant Shao Yang energy.

Dr. Kwon explained that those of Pancreotonia are, in a word, those who are always in a rush. These people, whether it be in walking or whatever, hate to fall behind others. They can't bear to sit still while there is work to be done, being of a diligent and active constitution. With a high degree of curiosity, they want to try anything, and if there is nothing for them to do, they will make something up. They have a quick eye for things, and thus among them are many artists.

A disease unique to those of Pancreotonia is vitiligo. There are also instances where infertility is seen among otherwise healthy people of this constitution.

- Beneficial food

Barley, Rice, Eggs, Wheat, Beans and nuts Red beans, Pork, Beef, Green Vegetables, All kinds of fishes and shellfishes, Persimmon, Pear, Melons, Strawberry, Cranberry and most Berries Banana, Vitamin E, Ice, Aloe vera, Mushrooms

5. Heat Tai Yin Constitution (Tai Yin type with Shao Yang quality)

Liver > Heart > Spleen > Kidney >Lung

Gall Bladder > Small Intestine >Stomach> Urinary Bladder > Large Intestine

AKA. Wood Yin body type. Cholecystonia.

Heat Taiyins have the strongest Liver and Gall bladder energy. Their Spleen and Stomach is relatively on the stronger side. The energy of Kidney and Urinary Bladder is on the weaker side, and their Lung and Large Intestine are the weakest.

They gain weight easily especially around the waist area. Their face is usually round or square, and their skin is relatively thick. With relatively stronger Earth Energy, their muscles have more resilience than Cold Taiyins. Some of Heat Taiyins are not heavy especially when they are young and exercise on a regular basis. However, with further interrogation, it is noticeable that they have pathological symptoms of weaker Lung or stronger Liver/GB, such as cough induced by wind cold or Gall stones. This body type can also develop high blood pressure, high cholesterol, or diabetes easily when they don't exercise enough or control their diet.

Dr. Kwon states that those of Cholecystonia are sensitive and are easily hurt by even the most innocent statements of others, and do not subsequently forget easily. Another notable characteristic is that they do well at sports involving throwing with the hand or kicking. When they take up sports like golf, soccer, or those that involve throwing, they are able to quickly surpass those who have been involved in such sports from even up to five years earlier. This is why considerations of constitution are important in choosing athletes. People of this constitution tend to have longer legs and arms and larger hands.

Among those of this body type, there are some serious alcoholics who seek alcohol even in their final, dying moments. Although those of other constitutions can develop disease through the excessive consumption of alcohol, they do not become as addicted as those of this body type. Alcoholism, therefore, is a sign that one is most likely of Cholecystonia.

• Beneficial food

Beef, Pork, Rice, Soybean, Wheat, Indian millet, Root Vegetables (radish, carrot, yam, lotus root, and taro) Coffee, Milk(warm), Garlic, Pumpkin or squash, Mushrooms, Sugar, All kinds of nuts (walnut, pecan, chestnut, pine-nut), Some fresh water fishes (eel, loach/mudfish), Alkaline beverages, Pear, Melons, Deer horn (herb), Squalene oil, Vitamin A and D

6. Cold Tai Yin Constitution (Tai Yin type with Shao Yin quality)

Liver > Kidney > Heart > Spleen > Lung

Gall Bladder> Urinary Bladder > Small Intestine >Stomach > Large Intestine

AKA.   Wood Yang body type. Hepatonia.

Cold Taiyins have the strongest Liver and Gall bladder energy. The next strongest are the Kidney and Urinary Bladder. Their Spleen and Stomach is relatively on the weaker side, and their Lung and Large Intestine are the weakest.

Cold Taiyins also gain weight easily especially around the waist area due to strong Liver energy. However, with relatively weaker Earth Energy, their muscles are rather flabby. They can develop high blood pressure, high cholesterol, or hypothyroidism easily when they don't exercise enough or control their diet.   Many of Cold Taiyins also suffer from allergic rhinitis or asthma.

According to Dr. Kwon, those people with this body type are reticent and taciturn, and do not speak much. They also become short of breath easily while singing. It is because they have small lungs, leading them to become tired more easily when talking a lot. Of course, with training they can learn to sing well, but generally the tone deaf fall into this category. In general, they are of large stature, and do not particularly like to argue over things.

A blood pressure of 170/80, which is seen as classic high blood pressure in others, is actually a normal, healthy state of those of Hepatonia. When that blood pressure fall s without any other symptoms, then the person's health will deteriorate and they will become fatigued. Later, this will lead to thrombus stroke, with the right side of the body being unusable and a speech impairment resulting. Of course this is only seen in instances of Hepatonia. In other constitutions, a blood pressure that is high would be seen as a dangerous condition.

Even for those of Hepatonia, one must of course be careful if the blood pressure exceeds 200. Should one of this constitution encounter a cerebral hemorrhage, then generally he or she will lose control of the left side of their body, while language will remain generally acceptable.

- Beneficial food

All kinds of Meats, Rice, Soybean, Wheat, Indian millet, Root Vegetables (radish, carrot, yam, lotus root, and taro) Coffee, Milk(warm), Garlic, Pumpkin or squash, Mushrooms, Sugar, Some fresh water fishes (eel, loach/mudfish), Alkaline beverages, Pear, Apple, Watermelon, Nuts (walnut, pecan, chestnut, pine-nut), Deer horn(herb), Ginseng, Vitamin A and D

7. Heat Tai Yang Constitution (Tai Yang type with Shao Yang quality)

Lung > Spleen > Heart > Kidney > Liver

Large Intestine>Stomach >Small Intestine >Urinary Bladder > Gall Bladder

AKA. Metal Yang body type. Pulmotonia.

Heat Taiyangs have the strongest Lung and Large Intestine energy. The next strongest are the Spleen and Stomach. Their Kidney and Urinary Bladder are relatively on the weaker side, and their Liver and Gall bladder are the weakest.

Heat Taiyangs usually thin, but their muscles are very well developed. Their facial characteristics are clearly defined and rugged. They have big shoulder area, but the lower portion from the waist down is weak.

As Dr. Kwon described in his paper, those of Pulmotonia are generally unrealistic, and do not like being in the spotlight. They have strong creativity, and are well suited to accomplishing their dream and desires.

- Beneficial food

All kinds of ocean fishes and shellfishes, Rice(White), Buckwheat, Mung beans, Mugwort, Cucumber, Eggplant, Cabbage, Lettuce, Green Vegetables, Bracken(fern), Dextrose, Cocoa/Chocolate, Banana, Strawberry, Peach, Cherry, Persimmon, Quince, Aloe vera, Ice, Dextrose injection, Vitamin E

8. Cold Tai Yang Constitution (Tai Yang type with Shao Yin quality)

Lung > Kidney> Spleen > Heart > Liver

Large Intestine>Urinary Bladder>Stomach>Small Intestine> Gall

Bladder

AKA. Metal Yin body type. Colonotonia.

Cold Taiyangs have the strongest Lung and Large Intestine energy. The next strongest are the Kidney and Urinary Bladder. Their Spleen and Stomach are relatively on the weaker side, and their Liver and Gall bladder are the weakest.

Cold Taiyangs usually thin, but their muscles are relatively well developed. Their facial characteristics are clearly defined and rugged. Due to the weak Liver and Spleen, alcohol can take a serious toll on their health.

Based on Dr. Kwon's theory, marathon runners tend to fall within Colonotonia. Although unable to run well for short distances, in long-distance runs when others begin to fall out from fatigue these people are able to get a second wind and complete the race to the end. They tend to become easily angered for reasons that they do not understand, but that is attributable to their eating meat.

Those of colonotonia are subject to Parkinson's Disease. By overindulging in meats, they can encounter both Parkinson's Disease and dementia. On the other hand, however, they do not contract myeloid leukemia.

- Beneficial food

Buckwheat, Rice(White), Dextrose, All kinds of ocean fishes and shellfishes(except oyster), Green Vegetables, Cucumber, Bracken(fern), Green seaweed, Grapes, Peach, Persimmon, Cherry, Pineapple, Strawberry, Mustard, Cocoa/Chocolate, Acanthopanax root bark, Swim, cold bath

Korean Constitutional Acupuncture Point Selection

Before identifying the formula of point selection, it is important to figure out the algorithm of the five elements. Assuming that all of you already learned the generating cycle and controlling cycle of the five elements from the curriculum of acupuncture school, the result of tonifying the Wood element would be as the picture below.

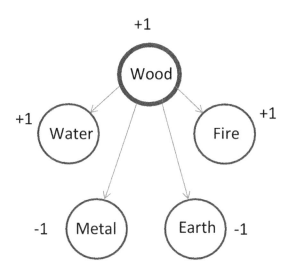

<The change of all the five elements when Wood is tonified>

The number is not an absolute value, but a relative one. To simplify the process, number 1 is used as an arbitrary value. When Wood is tonified, Water and Fire are tonified based on generating cycle, and Metal and Earth are sedated based on controlling relationship.

   A) Wood= +1   Water= +1   Fire= +1   Metal=-1   Earth =-1

Now let's think about the case where the Earth element is sedated. The result of Sedating the Earth element would be as the picture below.

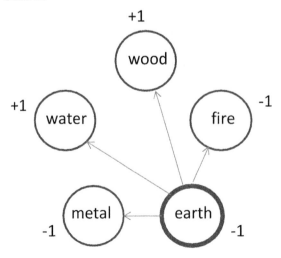

<The change of all the five elements when Earth is sedated>

When Earth is sedated, Fire and Metal are sedated based on generating cycle, and Water and Wood are sedated based on controlling relationship.

B) Wood= +1   Water= +1   Fire= -1   Metal=-1   Earth =-1

Then what would happen in the five element system when Wood is tonified and Earth is sedated at the same time in the clinical practice? You only need to add up A) and B).

A) + B)

Wood= +2   Water= +2   Fire= 0   Metal=-2   Earth =-2

This treatment could be applied for Heat Taiyangs or Heat Shaoyangs. (in other words, for Metal Yang or Earth yin)

Based on the algorithm explained above, the formula for Korean Constitutional Acupuncture can be deduced as below.

Point Selection for each Constitution I

	Heat Tai Yang / Cold Tai Yin	Cold Tai Yang / Heat Tai Yin	Cold Shao Yang / Heat Shao Yin	Heat Shao Yang / Cold Shao Yin
Basic formula	Sedate Metal Tonify Water (Tonify LV or GB)/ Tonify Metal Sedate Water (Sedate LV or GB)	Sedate Water Tonify Wood (Sedate LU or LI)/ Tonify Water Sedate Wood (Tonify LU or LI)	Sedate Earth Tonify Metal (Tonify KD or UB)/ Tonify Earth Sedate Metal (Sedate KD or UB)	Sedate Metal Tonify Water (Sedate SP or ST)/ Tonify Metal Sedate Water (Tonify SP or ST)
Inflammation or Antiviral formula	Sedate Metal Tonify Water (Sedate SP or ST)/ Tonify Metal Sedate Water	Sedate Water Tonify Wood (Tonify HT or SI)/ Tonify Water Sedate	Sedate Earth Tonify Metal (Sedate HT or SI)/ Tonify Earth Sedate Metal (Tonify HT or SI)	Sedate Metal Tonify Water (Tonify LV or GB)/ Tonify Metal Sedate Water (Sedate LV or GB)

	(Tonify SP or ST)	Wood (Sedate HT or SI)		
Mental formula	Sedate Earth Tonify Wood (PC or SJ)/ Tonify Metal Sedate Water (PC or SJ)	Sedate Water Tonify Wood (PC or SJ)/ Tonify Metal Sedate Fire (PC or SJ)	Sedate Fire Tonify Water (PC or SJ)/ Tonify Earth Sedate Metal (PC or SJ)	Sedate Metal Tonify Water (PC or SJ)/ Tonify Earth Sedate Wood (PC or SJ)
Inflammation or Vitality	Sedate Earth Tonify Wood (Sedate LU or LI)/ Tonify Earth Sedate Wood (Tonify LU or LI)	Sedate Metal Tonify Fire (Tonify LV or GB)/ Tonify Metal Sedate Fire (Sedate LV or GB)	Sedate Fire Tonify Water (Sedate SP or ST)/ Tonify Fire Sedate Water (Tonify SP or ST)	Sedate Earth Tonify Wood (Tonify KD or UB)/ Tonify Earth Sedate Wood (Sedate KD or UB)
Pain Control	Sedate Earth Tonify Wood (Tonify KD or UB)/ Tonify Earth Sedate Wood (Sedate KD or UB)	Sedate Metal Tonify Fire (Sedate KD or UB)/ Tonify Metal Sedate Fire (Tonify KD or UB)	Sedate Fire Tonify Water (Tonify LU or LI)/ Tonify Fire Sedate Water (Sedate LU or LI)	Sedate Earth Tonify Wood (Sedate LU or LI)/ Tonify Earth Sedate Wood (Tonify LU or LI)

Point Selection for each Constitution II

Yin Meridian	Heat Tai Yang / Cold Tai Yin	Cold Tai Yang / Heat Tai Yin	Cold Shao Yang / Heat Shao Yin	Heat Shao Yang / Cold Shao Yin
Basic formula I	LU8r LV4r KD10t LV8t / LU8t LV4t KD10r LV8r	KD10r LU5r LV1t LU11t / KD10t LU5t LV1r LU11r	SP3r KD3r LU8t KD7t / SP3t KD3t LU8r KD7r	LU8r SP5r KD10t SP9t / LU8t SP5t KD10r SP9r
Inflammation I	LU8r SP5r KD10t SP9t / LU8t SP5t KD10r SP9r /	KD10r HT3r LV1t HT9t / KD10t HT3t LV1r HT9r /	SP3r HT7r LU8t HT4t / SP3t HT7t LU8r HT4r /	LU8r LV4r KD10t LV8t / LU8t LV4t KD10r LV8r
Mental formula	PC7r PC9t / PC5t PC3r	PC3r PC9t / PC5t PC8r	PC8r PC3t / PC7t PC5r	PC5r PC3t / PC7t PC9r
Inflammation II	SP3r LU9r LV1t LU11t / SP3t LU9t LV1r LU11r	LU8r LV4r HT8t LV2t / LU8t LV4t HT8r LV2r	HT8r SP2r KD10t SP9t / HT8t SP2t KD10r SP9r	SP3r KD3r LV1t KD1t / SP3t KD3t LV1r KD1r
Pain Control	SP3r KD3r LV1t KD1t / SP3t KD3t LV1r KD1r	LU8r KD7r HT8t KD2t / LU8t KD7t HT8r KD2r	HT8r LU10r KD10t LU5t / HT8t LU10t KD10r LU5r	SP3r LU9r LV1t LU11t / SP3t LU9t LV1r LU11r

t=tonification, r=reduction

Point Selection for each Constitution III

Yang Meridian	Heat Tai Yang / Cold Tai Yin	Cold Tai Yang / Heat Tai Yin	Cold Shao Yang / Heat Shao Yin	Heat Shao Yang / Cold Shao Yin
Basic formula II	LI1r GB44r UB66t GB43t / LI1t GB44t UB66r GB43r	UB66r LI2r GB41t LI3t / UB66t LI2t GB41r LI3r	ST36r UB40r LI1t UB67t / ST36t UB40t LI1r UB67r	LI1r ST45r UB66t ST44t / LI1t ST45t UB66r ST44r
Antiviral formula	LI1r ST45r UB66t ST44t / LI1t ST45t UB66r ST44r	UB66r SI2r GB41t SI3t / UB66t SI2t GB41r SI3r	ST36r SI8r LI1t SI1t / ST36t SI8t LI1r SI1r	LI1r GB44r UB66t GB43t / LI1t GB44t UB66r GB43r
Mental formula	SJ10r SJ3t / SJ1t SJ2r	SJ2r SJ3t / SJ1t SJ6r	SJ6r SJ2t / SJ10t SJ1r	SJ1r SJ2t / SJ10t SJ3r
Vitality	ST36r LI11r GB41t LI3t / ST36t LI11t GB41r LI3r	LI1r GB44r SI5t GB38t / LI1t GB44t SI5r GB38r	SI5r ST40r UB66t ST44t / SI5t ST40t UB66r ST44r	ST36r UB40r GB41t UB65t / ST36t UB40t GB41r UB65r
Pain Control	ST36r UB40r GB41t UB65t / ST36t UB40t GB41r UB65r	LI1r UB67r SI5t UB60t / LI1t UB67t SI5r UB60r	SI5r LI5r UB66t LI2t / SI5t LI5t UB66r	ST36r LI11r GB41t LI3t / ST36t LI11t GB41r LI3r

				LI2r		

t=tonification, r=reduction

<The application of the formulas>

Basic formula: sprain or strain, all kinds of injury, or general pediatric disorder

Inflammation I: Inflammation of Yang organs. Disorders of esophagus, uterus, blood vessels, skin or membrane. Disorders of Ear, Nose, and Throat.

Inflammation II: Inflammation of Yin organs. Musculoskeletal disorders.

Antiviral formula: Infectious disease. Bacterial or viral disorders.

Vitality: Asthenia or adynamia. Gastroptosis, rectal prolapse, low appetite or chronic fatigue syndrome.

Mental formula: Neurosis, insomnia, or depression.

Additional body type and point selection

Dr. Yeom Taehwan, in his book <The treatment with constitutional acupuncture>[6], states that there exist 24 constitutions based on excess and deficiency of each 6 yang organs and 6 yin organs, which are Gall Bladder excess body type, Liver excess body type, Small Intestine excess body type, Triple burner excess body type, Heart excess body type, Pericardium excess body type, Stomach excess body type, Spleen excess body type, Large Intestine excess body type, Lung excess body type, Urinary Bladder excess body type, Kidney excess body type, Gall Bladder deficiency body type, Liver deficiency body type, Small Intestine deficiency body type, Triple burner deficiency body type, Heart deficiency body type, Pericardium deficiency body type, Stomach deficiency body type, Spleen deficiency body type, Large Intestine deficiency body type, Lung deficiency body type, Urinary Bladder deficiency body type, and Kidney deficiency body type.

As constitutional medicine study evolves, there has been many Korean medicine doctors who came up with their own theories of constitution with different number of body types. However, we have to keep in mind that all those stems from Dr. Lee's 4 constitutions and Dr. Kwon's 8 constitutions.

In my practice, most cases are treated with 8 constitutional point selection. About 5 percent of cases needed a variation that worked even better for them, which led me to add a couple more body types. These are also meaningful since one corresponds to Metal tonification and the other coincides with Earth Tonification in Sa

Am acupuncture (AKA four needle technique).

1. The Ninth Constitution

Liver > Heart > Kidney > Spleen > Lung

Gall Bladder> Small Intestine > Urinary Bladder >Stomach > Large Intestine

People with this body type have the strongest Liver and Gall bladder energy. The next strongest are the Heart and the small intestine. The next are Kidney and Urinary Bladder, which are still on the stronger side. Their Spleen and Stomach is relatively on the weaker side, and their Lung and Large Intestine are the weakest.

They are very similar to Cold Taiyins. Therefore, they also gain weight easily especially around the waist area due to strong Liver energy. However, with relatively weaker Earth Energy, their muscles are rather flabby. They can develop high blood pressure, high cholesterol, or hypothyroidism easily when they don't exercise enough or control their diet. They also tend to suffer from allergic rhinitis or asthma.

With stronger Fire energy, the lungs get even weaker causing more severe asthma and weight gain.

Point Selection

Basic formula: tonify earth, sedate fire

Sp3t Lu9t, Ht8r Lu10r

2. The Tenth Constitution

Kidney > Liver> Lung > Heart > Spleen

Urinary Bladder > Gall Bladder > Large Intestine > Small Intestine > Stomach

People with this body type have the strongest Kidney and UB energy. The second strongest are Liver and Gall Bladder. The next are the Lung and Large intestine, which are still on the stronger side. . Their Heart and Small intestine are relatively weaker, and their Spleen and Stomach are the weakest.

They are very similar to Cold Shaoyins. Therefore, they usually have a well-developed hip area and a less developed chest area. However, their Lung energy is also on the slightly stronger side, and the shoulder area is moderately well developed.

Point Selection

Basic formula: tonify fire, sedate wood

Ht8t Sp2t, Lv1r Sp1r

CHAPTER 2

JOSEON ACUPUNCTURE

Joseon is the name of a Korean dynastic kingdom that lasted from 1392 to 1897. While Chinese acupuncture was regarded inferior to herbal medicine in Qing Dynasty of China (1644-1840) and acupuncture gradually turned into a failure [7], there were two acupuncturists who developed unique approach of acupuncture in Joseon Dynasty of Korea.

One is 'Sa Ahm' who is a famous Buddhist monk and created the original Four Needle technique based on the traditional Asian philosophy of the five elements. Four Needle technique is already introduced in the curriculum of Acupuncture Schools in the US, and 8 constitutional acupuncture is also further developed based on this Four Needle technique utilizing the same five Shu points. Sa Ahm acupuncture is further discussed in Chapter 4.

The other is 'Heo Im'who was known for his contribution to the development of acupuncture and treated Seonjo (the 14th King of Joseon) and Gwanghaegun (the 15th King of Joseon). Later he wrote the book 'The Empirical Prescriptions of Acupuncture', which was republished in Japan in 1778 and was also introduced to Qing Dynasty of China in 1874 in the book of Zhen Jiu Ji Cheng written by Liao Runhong.

Dr. Heo's acupuncture technique has been further developed among other acupuncturists since Joseon Dynasty and this chapter will discuss the concept and methodology of acupuncture technique of Joseon.

The basic concept of Joseon acupuncture

Joseon acupuncture is the traditional Korean acupuncture technique that remained in existence and developed among Korean acupuncturists, not created by one person. It is more aggressive form of acupuncture treatment with thicker and longer needles that can be utilized in serious pain or illnesses including stroke, arthritis, spinal disc problems, or other musculosckeletal diseases.

In my clinical practice, I apply this technique to patients mostly over 50 years old when the treatment with the thinner needle doesn't seem to work due to more serious structural problems such as degeneration of joints or spinal discs.

These days needles with a diameter of 0.20mm – 0.25mm and a length of 13mm-40mm are generally used for most areas of the body.

In Joseon acupuncture, needles with a diameter of 0.5mm – 0.7mm and a length of 50mm- 120mm are used. The thicker needles are used because the thinner needles can be bent easily when they touch the interspinal ligament and make it difficult to go through the resistance.

However, in modern practice of Joseon acupuncture, needles with a diameter of 0.30mm-0.35mm and a length of 50mm-70mm are appropriate. This gauge still enables the needle to go through a fascia, a ligament or ligament adhesion, scar tissue, or hardened muscle tissue, and to reach the target area properly. For example, the points around cervical spine can be needled in a depth of 45mm with a 50mm length needle and the points around lumbar spine can be needled in a depth of 45mm-55mm with a 60mm needle to stimulate nervous system and ligaments effectively not damaging spinal cord.

Area of the body	Length of the needle	Depth of insertion
Neck area		40-45mm
face		10-45mm
Ear		10-45mm
Thoracic spine area	50mm	40-45mm
Shoulder area		30-45mm
Elbow area		20-45mm
Wrist area		10-45mm
Ankle area		30-45mm
Lumbar area	60mm	50-55mm

Knee area		50-55mm
Abdominal area		70-95mm
Femoral area	75mm-100mm	70mm
Gluteal area		50-70mm

<The depth of needle insertion depending on the area of the body>

The palpation of each acupuncture point is also very important in Joseon acupuncture because the interosseous points need to be found exactly between the bones and the points on the fibroids or tumor need to be inserted by a needle after finding exact location of the stagnation. After finding the exact point palpating the area with the thumb or index finger of the left hand, a needle can be inserted with the right hand with gentle manipulation of rotating the needle backward and forward, evenly and continuously.

 The article of Helene M. Langevin discussed the effects of acupuncture needling on the connective tissue, stating 'when acupuncture needle is rotated, collagen bundles adhere to the needle and wind around its shaft, creating a small whorl of collagen in the immediate vicinity of the needle within a few millimeter. [8] Not to mention the modern study on the needle manipulation, the efficacy of the manipulation has been highlighted in the history of acupuncture.

While manipulating the needle cautiously, it is crucial for both the acupuncturist and the patient to be able to feel the fishing Qi sensation. The fishing Qi sensation could be heavy, achy, numb, tingly, or like electric shock. Especially when the needle goes through the resistance of interspinal ligament and reaches the deepest layer, the patient can have a strong electric sensation. Also the sensation of the gentle manipulation ripples through the meridian or the whole body of the patient at times. Practitioners need to polish up the manipulation skill to achieve the fishing

Qi sensation by practicing on a carrot, a radish, or a roll of toilet paper.

In Joseon acupuncture, local points are mostly used. If L4 and L5 discs are degenerated causing pain, needles are inserted in L4 and L5 disc area. If there is a uterine fibroid, the points around the uterus and on the actual fibroid are needled.

In some cases, the scar tissue is too hard and thick to needle after surgery, the needle can be inserted after pulling the scar tissue with a left index finger. In case of bleeding, the area needs to be pressed with a cotton ball for about a minute. There could be healing signs before it gets better, such as leg pain or headaches after lumbar treatment, or joint pain after joint area treatment. It is important to let patients know this healing signs will be gone while treatments are continued.

SDN vs DDN

In the U.S., Dry needling or Intra-Muscular Stimulation (IMS) is introduced among physiotherapists by Dr. Chan Gunn. In the IMS studies, Superficial Dry Needling (SDN) and Deep Dry needling (DDN) were differentiated, and gave a theoretical statistical support for the deeper insertion of needles.

In the article of <Superficial versus Deep Dry Needling>[9], Peter Baldry states that SDN is not some new 20th century discovery, and that it was first described 2000 years ago in the book Huang Di Nei Jing. For DDN he gave an example of Chu's study as below.

'Chu has made a special study of a group of patients with clinical and electromyographic evidence of multi-level spondylotic radiculopathy, complicated by the secondary development of myofascial trigger point (MTrP) pain. 15-17 For this group she has developed a technique in which she obtains needle evoked multiple local twitch responses at the MTrP sites, a procedure she has called twitch-obtaining intramuscular stimulation (TOIMS). This method of carrying out DDN in this particular group of patients has proved very effective.'

However, Peter Baldry concludes his article by advocating SDN.

'It is my view that this and any of the other methods of carrying out DDN should be reserved for the relatively small number of patients in whom there is both MTrP and nerve root compression pain, and not used routinely for the treatment of uncomplicated MTrP nociceptive pain. My reason for saying this is because DDN gives rise to considerable treatment-evoked pain; it is liable to cause damage to neighboring structures, particularly blood vessels, and bleeding associated with the latter is responsible for the development of much troublesome posttreatment soreness.

For the reasons stated above I submit that SDN is the treatment of choice of the vast majority of patients who suffer from uncomplicated MTrP nociceptive pain, and that DDN should be reserved for the minority of those in whom there is concomitant MTrP and nerve root compression pain. '

First of all, Joseon acupuncture has been practiced among Korean Medicine doctors since 14th Century as a deep needling method, and I agree with Peter Baldry in that Deep needling can cause considerable treatment-evoked pain. That is why I only use this method for the patients who are over 50 years old and have degenerative disease of joints or spine. For this category of patient, superficial needling won't give much relief since the root of the problem is not treated. Only when you use this technique for the wrong category, it can give rise to more soreness. If you use it for the patients in the right category, it only creates benefit that Superficial needling or distal needling cannot provide. In addition to this, it is also important to abide by the recommendations from this book, for the thickness of the needles and the depth of insertion depending on the region of the body, for the maximum outcome of the treatment without damaging nervous system.

Huang Di Nei Jing was compiled over 2200 years ago during the Warring State period (475-221 BC)[10], and Superficial needling must have been enough to treat patients since the average life span of human being was much shorter than these days. In the modern society, as lifespan continues to increase and centenarians are becoming more common globally, the acupuncture treatment needs to be developed accordingly.

However, even when we add Joseon acupuncture as a deep needling technique in our practice, we should not overlook the fact that this deep needling technique has also been practiced since at least hundreds years ago.

The autonomic nervous system and Ren/Du meridians

In Joseon acupuncture, Du meridian points below the spinous processes of the vertebrae are also commonly used. For intractable diseases, allergies, or immunocompromised conditions, the points between T1 and L3 are applied to boost up our immunity by stimulating sympathetic nervous system and balancing with parasympathetic nervous system. The points on the cervical spine and Ren meridian of abdominal region are frequently utilized to reduce the stress by activating the parasympathetic nervous system and calming down the overactive sympathetic nervous system. These are also modern approach of Joseon acupuncture based on the anatomy of autonomic nervous system.

Based on the divisions of the autonomic nervous system, the cell bodies of the preganglionic axons of the sympathetic division are located in segments T1 through L3 of the lateral horn of the spinal cord. The parasympathetic division sends preganglionic neurons from the cranial area and the sacral area. This is why it is also known as the craniosacral division. The enteric nervous system (ENS) is sometimes referred to as the third division of the nervous system (central, peripheral, and enteric). This system is composed of a nerve plexus or a meshwork of fibers innervating the digestive tract from the esophagus to the distal colon. The ENS includes the myenteric plexus and the submucosal plexus which receive preganglionic fibers from the parasympathetic division and postganglionic fibers from the sympathetic division of the ANS. [11]

When it comes to the treatment utilizing the points on the Du meridian, it is also necessary to pay close attention to the efficacy related to the division and symptoms of autonomic nervous system.

<Cervical region>

C1	Supply blood to the head, pituitary gland, scalp, facial bone, brain, inner ear and middle ear, headaches, hypersensitivity, insomnia, hypertension, neurasthenia, sinus cold, migraine, forgetfulness, dizziness, chronic fatigue syndrome
C2	Eye, optic nerve, auditory nerve, vein, tongue, forehead, rhinitis, allergies, pain around eyes, pain in the ear, visual disturbance, phoria, deafness
C3	External ear, cheek, facial bone, teeth, neuralgia, neuritis, pimple, eczema
C4	Nose, Eustachian tube, lips, mouth, tenosynovitis, runny nose, hypoacusis, throat, tonsil
C5	Vocal cords, laryngitis, hoarseness
C6	Neck muscle, shoulder, tonsil, stiff neck, upper arm pain, tonsillitis, laryngitis, chronic cough
C7	Thyroid gland, bursa, elbow, common cold (Du14)

<Thoracic region>

T1	Hand, wrist, finger, elbow, lower arm, esophagus, bronchial asthma, cough, difficulty in breathing, rapid breathing,
T2	Heart, coronary artery

T3	Lung, bronchial tubes, pleura, chest, influenza, pleuritic, bronchitis, pneumonia
T4	Gall bladder, jaundice, shingles
T5	Liver, solar plexus, blood pressure, blood circulation, arthritis
T6	Stomach, digestion, heartburn
T7	Pancreas, stomach ulcer
T8	Spleen
T9	Kidneys, adrenal gland, rash
T10	Kidneys, chronic fatigue, arteriosclerosis, nephritis, pyelitis
T11	Kidneys, ureter, pimple, eczema
T12	Small intestine, lymph, rheumatoid arthritis, infertility

<Lumbar region>

L1	Large intestine, constipation, colitis, diarrhea, dysentery, enterocele,
L2	Appendix, abdomen, spasm of upper leg, breathing difficulty,
L3	Genital organs, uterus, urinary bladder, knee, menstrual cramp, irregular periods, lethargy
L4	Prostate gland, sciatic nerve, back pain, dysuria
L5	Lower leg, ankle, foot, poor circulation in the leg, swollen ankle, weak ankle, weak leg, cold foot, leg spasm

The empirical points of Joseon acupuncture

In the article <Dry needling gives you that 'twitch response'>, Melanie Plenda describes trigger point and the effect of the needling as below;

"As for trigger points, that's simply the tight painful knots that form when muscles are injured, or strained from repetitive motion. These trigger points are tender to the touch and can also cause pain that spreads to other parts of the body, called referred pain.
To release these knots, dry needling practitioners insert the needle in the trigger point and then move the needled in an up-and-down "pistoning" motion. Cyr said dry needling releases muscle tension, by causing tight muscles to twitch – or cramp – and then relax."[12]

Although it is true that acupuncture can relax the tightness of the muscles and release the knots as IMS practitioners describe, it is important to know that acupuncture can also strengthen and tighten the weakened muscles, ligaments, and fasciae. In the clinical practice, there are more cases of the latter especially in the geriatric diseases.

In this chapter, the commonly used points of Joseon acupuncture are discussed. When it comes to utilizing these points, it is recommended that practitioners keep in mind acupuncture has adaptogenic effect in immunity, hormones, and autonomic nervous system. In modern practices, the result of X-ray, MRI, ultrasound or CT can also help to decide where to put the needles. For example, if the pain is due to the herniated disc between L4 and L5, the needle should be inserted on Du3 which is located in the depression below the spinous process of the 4th lumbar vertebra.

1. Area of the Neck

- Du 16 (Fengfu 風附)

Location: 1 cun directly above the midpoint of the posterior hairline, directly below the external occipital protuberance, in the depression between m. trapezius of both sides.
Indications: Influenza, sore throat, headaches, sinus congestion, epistaxis, aphasia, hemiplegia, mental disorders, stoke
Method: Puncture perpendicularly 20-40mm with a 0.30x50mm needle with gentle manipulation of rotating the needle backward and forward, evenly and continuously.

- Du 14 (Dazhui 大椎)

Location: Below the spinous process of the seventh cervical vertebra, approximately at the level of the shoulders.
Indications: bronchitis, cough, common cold, neck pain and rigidity, back pain and stiffness, epilepsy, febrile disease, malaria, asthma, disc problems in the neck
Method: Puncture obliquely upward 45mm with a 0.30x50mm needle with gentle manipulation of rotating the needle backward and forward, evenly and continuously.

- Du 12 (Shenzhu 身柱)

Location: Below the spinous process of the third thoracic

vertebra.

Indications: bronchitis, cough, asthma, pneumonia, mental disorder, pain and stiffness of the back, epilepsy, neurasthenia

Method: Puncture obliquely upward 45mm with a 0.30x50mm needle with gentle manipulation of rotating the needle backward and forward, evenly and continuously.

· GB20 (Fengchi 風池)

Location: In the depression between the upper portion of m. sternocleidomastoideus and m. trapezius, on the same level with Du16.

Indications: Insomnia, headaches, vertigo, pain and stiffness of the neck, blurred vision, glaucoma, tinnitus, convulsion, epilepsy, febrile disease, common cold, nasal obstruction, rhinorrhea

Method: Puncture 30-45mm toward nose with a 0.30x50mm needle with gentle manipulation of rotating the needle backward and forward, evenly and continuously.

· GB21 (Jianjing 肩井)

Location: On the shoulder, directly above the nipple, at the midpoint of the line connecting Dazhui (Du14) and the and the acromion, at the highest point of the shoulder.

Indication: Disc problems in the cervical spine, pain and rigidity of the neck, pain in the shoulder and back, motor impairment of the arm, apoplexy, difficult labor

Method: Puncture perpendicularly 10mm with a 0.30x50mm needle with gentle manipulation of rotating the needle backward and forward, evenly and continuously.

2. Area of the Shoulder

· LI16 (Jugu 巨骨)

Location: In the upper aspect of the shoulder, in the

depression between the acromial extremity of the clavicle and the scapular spine.

Indication: Pain and motor impairment of the upper extremities, pain in the shoulder and back.

Method: Puncture perpendicularly 20-45mm with a 0.30x50mm needle with gentle manipulation of rotating the needle backward and forward, evenly and continuously.

- Ext23 (Jianqian 肩前)

Location: Midway between the end of the anterior axillary fold and LI15

Indication: Pain in the shoulder and arm, paralysis of the upper extremities

Method: Puncture perpendicularly 20-45mm with a 0.30x50mm needle with gentle manipulation of rotating the needle backward and forward, evenly and continuously.

- Extra point Jianzhong 肩中 (not listed in CAM)

Location: Inferior to the acromion, on the upper portion of m. deltoideus, the point is in the depression midpoint between LI15 and SI10.

Indication: Shoulder pain and stiffness

Method: Puncture perpendicularly 45mm with a 0.30x50mm needle with gentle manipulation of rotating the needle backward and forward, evenly and continuously.

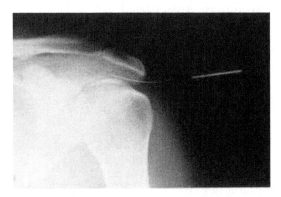

<X-ray of Jianzhong inserted 45mm with a 50mm needle>

- LI11 (Quchi 曲池)

Location: When the elbow is flexed, the point is in the depression at the lateral end of the transverse cubital crease midway between Lu5 and the lateral epicondyle of the humerus.

Indications: motor impairment of upper extremities, abdominal pain, vomiting, diarrhea

Method: Puncture perpendicularly 45mm with a 0.30x50mm needle with gentle manipulation of rotating the needle backward and forward, evenly and continuously.

3. Area of the Leg

- St36 (Zusanli 足三里)

Location: 3 cun below St35, one finger-breadth (middle finger) from the anterior border of the tibia.

Indication: Gastric pain, vomiting, hiccup, abdominal distention, borborygmus, diarrhea, constipation, enteritis, aching of the knee joint and leg, beriberi, edema, cough, asthma, emaciation due to general deficiency, indigestion, apoplexy, hemiplegia, dizziness, insomnia, mania

Method: Puncture perpendicularly 55mm with a 0.35x60mm needle with gentle manipulation of rotating the needle backward and forward, evenly and continuously.

- Extra point Xizhong (膝中)

Location: The point is in the depression between medial and lateral Xiyan, locating the point with the knee flexed.

Indications: Knee pain, knee sprain especially of anterior cruciate ligament

Method: Puncture perpendicularly 55mm with a

0.35x60mm needle with gentle manipulation of rotating the needle backward and forward, evenly and continuously.

- Extra 36 (Xiyan 膝眼)

Location: A pair of points in the two depressions, medial and lateral to the patellar ligament, locating the point with the knee flexed. These two points are also termed medial and lateral Xiyan respectively. Lateral Xiyan overlaps with ST35.
Indications: Knee pain, weakness of the lower extremities
Method: Puncture perpendicularly 55mm with a 0.35x60mm needle with gentle manipulation of rotating the needle backward and forward, evenly and continuously.

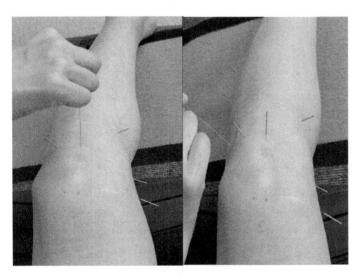

<Xiyan points (2 points) being inserted 55mm with a 60mm needle> -all other needles are 15mm

- UB40 (Weizhong 委中)

Location: Midpoint of the transverse crease of the popliteal fossa, between the tendons of m. biceps femoris and m. semitendinosus.

Indications: sprain or strain of the low back, Low back pain, motor impairment of hip joint, contracture of tendons in the popliteal fossa, motor impairment of lower extremities

Method: Puncture perpendicularly 30-55mm with a 0.35x60mm needle with gentle manipulation of rotating the needle backward and forward, evenly and continuously.

4. Area of the Back

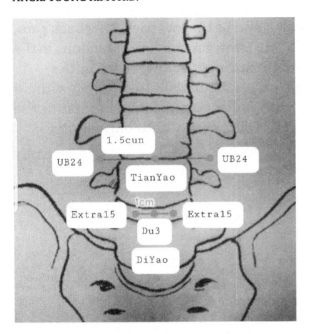

- UB24 (Qihaishu 氣海俞)

Location: 1.5 cun lateral to the Du meridian, at the level of the lower border of the spinous process of the third lumbar vertebra.

Indications: Low back pain, dysmenorrhea

Method: Puncture perpendicularly 40-55mm with a 0.35x60mm needle with gentle manipulation of rotating the needle backward and forward, evenly and continuously.

- Extra 15 (Huatuojiaji 華佗夾脊)

Location: A group of 34 points on both sides of the spinal column, 0.5 cun lateral to the lower border of each spinous process from the first thoracic vertebra to the fifth lumbar vertebra. (In the picture above, only one pair of this extra points are used.)

Indications: Low back pain, motor impairment of lower extremities

Method: Puncture perpendicularly 40-55mm with a 0.35x60mm needle with gentle manipulation of rotating the needle backward and forward, evenly and continuously.

- Extra point Tianyao (天要 not listed in CAM)

Location: Below the spinous process of the third lumbar vertebra.

Indications: Low back pain, disc problems

Method: Puncture perpendicularly 50-55mm with a 0.35x60mm needle with gentle manipulation of rotating the needle backward and forward, evenly and continuously.

- Du 3 (Yaoyangguan 要陽關)

–also called Renyao(人要) in Joseon acupuncture

Location: Below the spinous process of the fifth lumbar vertebra.

Indications: Low back pain, impotence, motor impairment, numbness and pain of lower extremities, pain in the lumbosacral region.

Method: Puncture perpendicularly 50-55mm with a 0.35x60mm needle with gentle manipulation of rotating the needle backward and forward, evenly and continuously.

- Extra point Diyao (地要 not listed in CAM)

Location: Below the spinous process of the fifth lumbar vertebra.

Indications: Low back pain, disc problems

Method: Puncture perpendicularly 50-55mm with a 0.35x60mm needle with gentle manipulation of rotating the needle backward and forward, evenly and continuously.

CHAPTER 3

SA AHM
ACUPUNCTURE

Introduction

Sa Ahm was a famous Buddhist monk who lived in Joseon dynasty and created the original Four Needle technique based on the traditional Asian philosophy of the five elements. Sa Ahm acupuncture is already introduced as Four Needle technique in the curriculum of Acupuncture Schools in the US, and 8 constitutional acupuncture is also further developed based on this Four Needle technique utilizing the same five Shu points.

Sa Ahm acupuncture was originally described in a manuscript that is estimated to be published at some point between 1644 and 1742, in the middle of the Joseon dynasty. The principle of combining five shu points is based on the theory of Nan-jing. The treatment and diagnosis concepts in Sa ahm acupuncture were mainly influenced by Dongui Bogam and Chimgoogyeong-heombang ('The Empirical Prescriptions of Acupuncture'). The basic characteristic of combining five shu points in Sa Ahm acupuncture is the selection of the tonification and sedation points along the self-meridian and other meridians based on creation and governor relationships.

Sa Ahm acupuncture, which is one of the original therapeutic modalities representing traditional Korean medicine, is a unique treatment method that has a different origin than the modalities from China and Japan. The basic characteristic of combining five shu points in Sa Ahm acupuncture is the selection of the tonification and sedation points along the self-meridian and other meridians based on creation and governor relationships. In China, five element acupuncture, tonification, and sedation points along only the self-meridian are selected. Japanese meridian therapy added source point, connecting point, cleft point, alarm point, and transport point on the basis of Korea Sa Ahm acupuncture conception of the combined five shu points.[13]

The original manuscript that described Sa ahm acupuncture is estimated to have been published between 1644 and 1742, in the middle of the Joseon dynasty. Because Chimgoogyeong-heombang ('The Empirical Prescriptions of Acupuncture'), which was published in 1644, is quoted in the manuscript of Sa ahm acupuncture, the publication period of the Sa Ahm acupuncture manuscript can be estimated to be after 1644. After 1742, Gy-san's clinical experience was added to the original manuscript of Sa Ahm acupuncture, that is, Gyeongjeyogyeol (Essential Rhymes on Acupuncture and Moxibustion by Master Sa Ahm). This is the oldest existing manuscript associated with Sa Ahm acupuncture. The physiology, pathology, and disease identification sections of Sa Ahm were handed down to its disciples, but the clinical experience section of Gy-san coexists in the currently published Sa Ahm acupuncture-related books.

Viscera/bowel-based acupuncture was developed in Chimgoogyeong-heombang ('The Empirical Prescriptions of Acupuncture'), with integration of the meridian/exterior theory with the viscera manifestation theory, which in turn provided various methods for viscera diagnosis. Viscera identification became the basis of Sa Ahm acupuncture treatment.

The Dongui Bogam (Treasured Mirror of Eastern Medicine) contains the following phrase: "One acupuncture needle in all the diseases, up to within four acupuncture needles, acupuncture on the whole body is not a good idea." This phrase represents the characteristics of the traditional Korean acupuncture method. In this context, Sa Ahm acupuncture treated the disease within four acupuncture points. Further, an acupuncture method based on the five element principles is presented in the acupuncture section of the Dongui Bogam. The idea of treating a disease derived from viscera/bowel dysfunction by using five shu points influenced Sa Ahm acupuncture.[14]

Basic Theories

The following phrase is taken from the 69th chapter of Nan-jing: "In the case of depletion, fill the respective mother, in the case of repletion, drain the respective child, one must fill the first and then drain afterward." Gao-Wu, of the Ming Dynasty of China (1519 A.D.), was the first acupuncturist to describe the use of tonification and sedation points along the self-meridian by using the five shu points according to the 69th issue of Nan-Jing. Zhang Shi Xian advocated the use of five shu points in other meridians in Jiao Zheng Tu Zhu Nan Jing (Illustrated note of Classic of Difficult Issues). On the basis of Gao-Wu and Zhang Shi Xian treatment, Sa Ahm added the role of the governor. This notion originated from the 50th and 75th chapters of Nan-Jing.

Chapter 50

Among the illnesses are the depletion, repletion, destroyer, weakness, and regular evils. How are they distinguished? Those (illnesses) coming from behind represent a depletion evil. Those coming from ahead represent a repletion evil. Those coming from what cannot be overcome represent a destroyer evil. Those coming from what can be overcome rep-resent a weakness evil. If the respective depot is afflicted from within itself, it represents a regular evil.

Chapter 75

If East is excess and West is deficient, sedate the South and tonify the North.

In Sa Ahm acupuncture, the relationship with the governor is important, as is the relationship between the mother and son. The governor is sedated under the condition of deficiency and is tonified under the condition of excess.

The basic rules are those of the creation and governor relationships. In the case of insufficiency of any meridian, the mother points of its mother and its own meridians should be tonified and the governor points of its governor and its own meridians should be sedated. For example, the following is applied if the lung meridian is diagnosed as deficient: earth tonification, lung meridian-earth point LU9 and spleen meridian-earth point SP3 and fire sedation, lung meridian-fire point LU10, and heart meridian-fire point HT8. The other meridians follow the same rule, as described above.

In the case of the excess of any meridians, the governor points of its governor and its own meridians should be tonified and the son points of its son and its own meridians should be sedated. For example, the following is applied if the lung meridian is diagnosed to be excessive: fire tonification, lung meridian-fire point LU10, and heart meridian-fire point HT8 and water sedation, lung meridian-water point LU5, and kidney meridian-water point KI10.

Please refer to the Table 1.

Table 1

Sa Ahm's combination of five shu points for deficiency and excess of the meridians.

Meridian	Deficiency				Excess			
	Tonify		Sedate		Tonify		Sedate	
Lung	SP3	LU9	HT8	LU10	HT8	LU19	KI10	LU5
Large intestine	ST36	LI11	SI5	LI5	SI5	LI5	BL66	LI2
Stomach	SI5	ST41	GB41	ST43	GB41	ST43	LI1	ST45
Spleen	HT8	SP2	LR1	SP1	LR1	SP1	LU8	SP5
Heart	LR1	HT9	KI19	HT3	KI19	HT3	SP3	HT7
Small intestine	GB41	SI3	BL66	SI2	BL66	SI2	ST36	SI8
Bladder	LI1	BL67	ST36	BL54	ST36	BL54	GB41	BL65
Kidney	LU8	KI7	SP3	KI3	SP3	KI3	LR1	KI1
Pericardium	LR1	PC9	KI10	PC3	KI10	PC3	SP3	PC7
Triple Burner	GB41	SJ3	BL66	SJ2	BL66	SJ2	ST36	SJ10
Gall bladder	BL66	GB43	LI1	GB44	LI1	GB44	SI5	GB38
Liver	KI10	LR8	LU8	LR4	LU8	LR4	HT8	LR2

Another simple but rarely used one is coldness-fire acupuncture treatment derived from the deficiency-excess acupuncture treatment. For cold symptoms, the fire points of its own and the fire meridians are tonified and the Water points of its own and the water meridians are sedated. For heat symptoms, the water points of its own and the water meridians are tonified and the fire points of its own and the fire meridians are sedated.

Please refer to the Table 2.

Table 2

Sa Ahm's combination of five shu points for cold and heat symptoms of the meridians.

Meridians	Cold				Fire			
	Tonify		Sedate		Tonify		Sedate	
Lung	HT8	LU10	LU5	KI10	LU5	KI10	SP3	LU9
Large intestine	SI5	ST41	LI2	BL66	LI2	BL66	SI5	ST41
Stomach	ST41	SI5	ST44	BL66	ST44	BL66	ST36	BL54
Spleen	SP2	HT8	SP9	KI10	SP9	KI10	SP3	KI3
Heart	HT8	KI2	HT3	KI10	HT3	KI10	HT8	KI2
Small intestine	SI5	BL60	SI2	BL66	SI2	BL66	SI8	ST36
Bladder	SI5	BL60	SI2	BL66	SI2	BL66	ST36	BL54
Kidney	HT8	KI2	KI10	HT3	KI10	HT3	SP3	KI3
Pericardium	HT8	PC8	PC3	HT3	PC3	HT3	SP3	PC7
Triple Burner	SJ6	BL60	SJ2	BL66	SJ2	BL66	SJ6	BL60
Gall bladder	GB38	SI5	GB43	BL66	GB43	BL66	BL54	GB34
Liver	LR2	HT8	KI10	LR8	KI10	LR8	LR3	SP3

Among the clinical case studies of Sa ahm, 85% used either a tonification or a sedation formula, whereas 15% used variations of the tonification and the sedation formulae. Sa Ahm treatment primarily focuses on the viewpoints of deficiency-excess symptoms rather than cold-heat symptoms.[15]

Sa Ahm acupuncture is based on the traditional concepts of yin-yang, five elements, ZangFu (viscera and bowels), qi, and meridians. Sa Ahm acupuncture treatment cannot be separated from these viewpoints. In particular, it involves the application of five shu points according to the creation and control cycles of the five-element theory. Therefore, the combination of acupoints in Sa Ahm is easier to understand from the perspective of traditional medicine.

The meridian is divided into three parts: the arm or foot, three yin and yang, and six ZangFu parts. A total of 24 deficiency and excess symptoms, with 24 coldness and fire symptoms, exist across the 12 meridians, but the diagnostic criteria related to these symptoms are too ambiguous for selecting a correct meridian. Except for the regular 48-treatment protocol, the treatment strategies are largely variable. Efforts were made to produce Sa Ahm treatments that are more effective by including other acupoints, with the main points firmly based on the regular pattern. However, because the explanation regarding acupoint selection is very brief or elided, applying Sa Ahm acupuncture in the clinic is difficult.

As described in <A Modern Clinical Approach of the Traditional Korean Sa Ahm Acupuncture>, various Korean scholars have suggested different methods for applying Sa Ahm acupuncture in the clinic. Lee[16] proposed a diagnostic system by comparing pulse examination, whereas Kim[17] proposed a symptom-based diagnosis. Cho[18] established visceral pattern identification for providing easy access to Sa Ahm acupuncture by analyzing

Neijing (Internal Classic), Nan-jing (Classic of Difficult Issues), and Yixuerumen (Introduction to Medicine). Moreover, Kwon[19] studied constitutional acupuncture, and Kim[20] reviewed the mind-based aspect of Sa Ahm acupuncture.

Based on my clinical experience, diagnosing by physical appearance combined with identifying symptoms showed the highest efficacy. It is definitely useful to explain it in the same context as constitutional acupuncture approach. However, identifying constitution by pulse examination is not recommended since it is too ambiguous. It is crucial to pay attention to the genius of Dr. Lee jema and the meaning of 'Sasang(四相)', which is the four images. The 'image' of physical appearance is definitely the key to identify constitution along with other traits. The details of how to identify constitution is described in the chapter 1.

In terms of identifying symptoms in utilizing Sa Ahm acupuncture, the concept of 'the six energy(六氣)' can be adopted from Nei-Jing.

Chapter 68

The six influences of cold, fire, dryness, dampness, heat, and wind are referred to as the ben or primary aspect. The three yang and the three yin channels of taiyang, shaoyang, yangming, taiyin, shaoyin, and jueyin are referred to as the biao or secondary aspect of the six influences. The ben originates in the cosmos while the biao manifests on earth.[21]

The associations of five element, six energy, and three yin three yang meridians are as below.

Jueyin Wind Wood

Shaoyin Imperial Fire

Taiyin Damp Earth

Shaoyang Ministerial Fire

Yangming Dry Metal

Taiyang Cold Water

As we go over each meridian, the application of this concept will be introduced. This also could be understood in the context of Ba Gua, the eight trigrams. Please refer to Table 3.

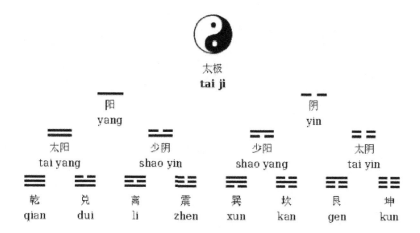

Table 3

Eight Trigram								
	☷	☶	☵	☴	☳	☲	☱	☰
name	Kun Earth	Gen Mountain	Kan Water	Xun Wind	Zhen Thunder	Li Fire	Dui Lake	Qian Heaven
meridian	Ren	Yang-ming	Tai-yang	Jue-yin	Shao-yang	Shao-yin	Tai-yin	Du
6 climatic energy		Dry-ness	Cold	Wind	Minist-erial Fire	Mona-rch Fire	Damp-ness	

In actual insertion of needles, there are some characteristics are noticeable in Sa Ahm acupuncture. Men are needled on the left side and women on the right. It is only done on One side of the body, usually on the healthy side. Needling direction tonifies when flowing with direction of meridian and sedates against the direction of meridian. Rotating the needle clockwise tonifies, and counter clockwise sedates. Inserting the needle while patient exhales tonifies, while inhale sedates. Closing the hole after needle withdrawal tonifies, while keeping hole open sedates. Slow insertion fast withdrawal tonifies, fast insertion, slow withdrawal sedates.[22]

Having said that, it varies depending on the providers in ways of practicing the techniques of Sa Ahm.

The case studies of this chapters are mainly extracted from Dr. Kim Hongkyung's 'Revolution of Oriental Medicine'.

Hand Yangming Large Intestine Meridian

LI tonification: ST36t, LI11t, SI5r, LI5r

LI sedation: SI5t, LI5t, UB66r, LI2r

LI cooling: UB66t, LI2t, SI5r, LI5r

LI warming: SI5t, LI5t, UB66r, LI2r

1. Indications

Hand Yangming LI meridian has dry energy from metal element. Yangming dry energy can dry the dampness. LI tonification also has cooling function since the tonification of LI is composed of the points of tonifying earth (mother) and the points of sedating fire (grandmother). LI meridian is connected to Large Intestine organ; therefore, it can be used for LI diseases as well as pain on LI channel.

Yangming prevents and stops the internal wind. It is said that numbness on the second finger indicates that wind stroke may occur within three years. That means Yangming deficiency may lead to wind stroke, hence tonification of Yangming dryness can prevent wind stroke. Obesity is considered due to dampness accumulation It is said that obese people are more vulnerable to wind stroke because dampness can cause qi stagnation and heat which turns into stagnated fire and causes wind stroke. Yangming dryness can prevent internal wind by drying up the dampness.

With LI tonification, Bi syndrome, especially damp Bi, can be treated. Obesity, frontal headaches, nasal obstruction, nasal discharge, scrofula, and skin disease due to damp heat can be treated as well.

By selecting LI meridian, Large intestine diseases can be treated along with abdominal distention, leukorrhea, shoulder pain, toothaches, and lower back pain due to dampness.

2. Case studies

- A 56 year old female had a pain around umbilicus which was accompanied by diarrhea She also complained of pain in medial malleolus, headaches, dizziness, and stiffness in her neck. She had a history of choledocholithotomy. She was keen and very irritable. Diarrhea ha significantly reduced after 2 treatments on hand Yangming Large Intestine tonification and foot Shaoyang Gall Bladder sedation.

- A 27 year old male, 5'8", 180lbs, suffered from chronic fatigue, lassitude during day time, no appetite, and indigestion for the past 3months. His limbs were cold and he often had diarrhea. Pulse was slow. Treatments were given on hand Yangming Large Intestine tonification. He felt refreshed after the treatment and after 1 week most of the symptoms disappeared.

- A 52 year old male suffered from numbness, pain in the arm and occasional insect crawling sensation in the leg joints. Eliminating dampness seemed to be an appropriate treatment for him. In fact, he was completely cured after a few treatments on hand Yangming Large Intestine tonification.

Foot Yangming Stomach Meridian

ST tonification: SI5t, ST41t, GB41r, ST43r

ST sedation: GB41t, ST43t, LI1r, ST45r

ST cooling: UB66t, ST44t, SI5r, ST41r

ST warming: ST41t, SI5t, UB66r, ST44r

1. Indications

Foot Yangming Stomach meridian has dry energy from earth element. Dry energy dries dampness Stomach and Spleen have opposite energy flow. Spleen Qi goes up while Stomach Qi goes down. Therefore, tonification of stomach meridian can pull rebellious Qi down and uprising Shaoyang fire as well. Tonification of Stomach is composed of tonification of fire points (mother) and sedation of wood points (grandmother), so Stomach tonification can warm the inside as well as pull down and clear the Shaoyang fire.

With Stomach tonification, anxiety, headaches with dizziness, and swelling/pain of the eyes can be treated by pulling down the uprising Shaoyang fire. Nausea and vomiting also can be treated by pulling down rebellious Qi.

With its Yangming energy, it can prevent and stop the internal wind. With its drying function, it can threat damp-Bi syndrome in four limbs which are governed by the earth.

Stomach tonification also can be used for indigestion, abdominal distention, gastric ulcer, and diarrhea due to dampness.

2. Case studies

- A 60-year-old female, slightly obese, suffered from a lingering cold for a month. She had an indigestion which has started after taking an over-the-counter medicine during early stage of common cold. Distention and bloating sensation were gone after one treatment on foot Yangming Stomach tonification. This is due to action of dry energy of Yangming and improvement of the Stomach function of transform and transport of dampness.

- A male patient in his mid-thirties, suffered from lower back pain and numbness in the limbs. He has slightly yellow and dull complexion. One peculiar symptom was that he had excessive amount of eye wax for years. His pulse was rapid. Treatments of foot Yangming Stomach tonification were done to promote circulation and eliminate damp. After a couple treatments the symptom of eye wax was completely gone.

- A 60-year-old female who is overweight, suffered from edema and knee pain. Improvement, to a certain extent, was observed after foot Yangming Stomach tonification.

- A 29-year-old male, 5'9" and 143lbs, suffered from nausea, vomiting, and diarrhea after having a common cold for 2 weeks. He had an abdominal pain which was worse if it was accompanied by diarrhea. The pain was alleviated with warmth and pressure. However, the pain was gradually aggravated with time. He experienced more frequent diarrhea as time passed. Tongue had a white coating and pulse was slow. There was no thirst. Diarrhea ceased after 3-4 treatments of foot Yangming Stomach tonification.

- A 50-year-old male who is slightly overweight, suffered from indigestion, right knee pain, food stagnation after having pork. He also had abdominal pain which is relieved after bowel movement. He was completely cured after one treatment of foot Yangming Stomach tonification.

- A 40-year-old male, 5'8" and 165lbs, had been out of country for one and a half year, and gained about 7lbs. He had history of lumbar disc problem which recurred recently. He also had been diagnosed by his ENT doctor that his auditory tube had been blocked. It had aggravated gradually. These days he had suffered from hearing and was unable to stand pressure difference while he was on board in airplane. He had 3 treatments of draining water from auditory tube so far due to this problem. There also had been stubborn phlegm in the body since his childhood. Ear problem had cured after 6 treatments of foot Yangming Stomach tonification.

Hand Taiyin Lung Meridian

LU tonification: SP3t, LU9t, HT8r, LU10r

LU sedation: HT8t, LU10t, KD10r, LU5r

LU cooling: KD10t, LU5t, HT8r, LU10r

LU warming: HT8t, LU10t, KD10r, LU5r

1. Indications

Taiyin Lung meridian has damp energy from metal element. Taiyin damp energy moistens dryness. Dry heat, from Yin deficiency, can be treated with Taiyin Lung tonification. Lung tonification is composed with tonification of earth points and sedation of fire points, so it also has cooling function. Lung meridian is connected with Lung organ and controls skin, therefore Lung disease and skin diseases can be treated with Lung channel treatment.

Lung governs Qi, so Lung tonification can tonify the Qi deficiency.

Lung tonification can treat Lung organ related diseases such as common cold, cough, asthma, and pulmonary tuberculosis.

Skin belongs to the Lung system; therefore, skin disease can be treated with Lung meridian. Also, Taiyin damp energy can treat dryness as well as heat from yin deficiency.

With Taiyin Lung tonification, eye disease from dry heat, especially from Lung dry heat, can be treated. (ex. Redness of sclera) Nasal obstruction, caused by dryness in respiratory system, also can be treated. Wei syndrome, caused by Lung dry heat, can be treated as well.

2. Case studies

- A 9-year-old girl, normal physique, had lingering cold for 3 months. She had dry cough which had now become chronic. She was diagnosed with 'stiffened vocal cord' by M.D. and told to wait until it softens. After sleep, in the morning, even a slight conversation made her lose her voice, and singing seemed almost impossible. To aid flexibility and moistening function, a treatment was rendered with hand Taiyin Lung tonification. The next morning her voice had got much clearer, and after 3 treatments it showed a significant improvement.

- A male patient of his early 50's suffered from stuffy nose which accompanied by yellow nasal discharge and frontal headaches for a few years. He also had a nasal voice. He had many treatments previously for the same problem, but they only worked temporarily. A treatment of hand Taiyin Lung tonification was rendered since the nose is the window of lung and the Lung governs Qi. After 3 to 4 treatments symptoms were gradually improved.

45. A 61-year-old male, 150lbs and 5'6", had suffered from chronic cough which was accompanied by watery white phlegm. The symptoms were worse at night. He had a poor appetite and diarrhea with 3-4

times of bowel movements a day. His complexion was dull yellow. Tongue had sticky coating and pulse was slippery. His symptoms were considered to be constrained cold in the Lung. Warming technique of Hand Taiyin Lung was very effective on this case.

Foot Taiyin Spleen Meridian

SP tonification: HT8t, SP2t, LV1r, SP1r

SP sedation: LV1t, SP1t, SP5r, LU8r

SP cooling: KD10t, SP9t, HT8r, SP2r

SP warming: HT8t, SP2t, KD10r, SP9r

1. Indications

Taiyin Spleen meridian has damp energy from earth element. Spleen regulates dampness and damp energy can moisten dryness. Spleen Qi transforms and transports dampness all over the body. Therefore, Spleen Qi deficiency can cause damp accumulation and Spleen tonification can regulate dampness. Also, Spleen tonification has warming function since Spleen tonification is composed of wood sedation and fire tonification. Spleen meridian is connected to Spleen organ, so it can be used for any Spleen related diseases.

With Spleen tonification, overall dryness and partial dampness can be treated. It can be used when Spleen failed to transform and transport the dampness due to Spleen Qi deficiency. Spleen tonification can tonify spleen Qi and spread damp accumulation.

Food related diseases also can be treated with Spleen tonification, such as food poisoning, food stagnation, and indigestion.

Spleen tonification can treat Edema due to Spleen deficiency. This kind of edema is caused by impaired transforming and transporting function of Spleen.

It can also treat Diabetes since Diabetes belongs to Spleen disorder.

Spleen governs four limbs, so Spleen tonification can treat disorders of four limbs.

Low appetite, constipation, and diarrhea can be regulated by Spleen as well.

2. Case studies

- A 42-year-old male, 5'5", 92lbs, had extremely cold extremities so he could not even sit on a cold floor. He also had indigestion and constipation. He had suffered from above symptoms for the past 6 years and recently lost another 6lbs. Slight improvement was observed after a few treatments with foot Taiyin spleen tonification.

- A 25-year-old male suffered from alternating vomiting and diarrhea form 2 hours after having a cold noodle. Since that incident, he felt very tired and dizzy. He vomited right away when food was ingested. His complexion was pale. Symptoms were completely cured after treatment of foot Taiyin Spleen tonification.

48. A 34-year-old male, 5'5" and 135lbs, had congenital mental weakness. His speech was inarticulate. His complexion was pale and pulse was weak. His

extremities were very cold. He usually had a light meal and often suffered from indigestion. Deficient cold in spleen and Stomach seemed to be an origin of such indigestion. Foot Taiyin Spleen tonification and PC9 were used. After 2 treatments, indigestion had significantly improved and even his extremities had gotten warmer than before. This was focused on aiding Spleen for smooth channel flow throughout the limbs.

Hand Taiyang Small Intestine Meridian

SI tonification: SI3t, GB41t, SI2r, UB66r

SI sedation: SI2t, UB66t, SI8r, ST36r

SI cooling: UB66t, SI2t, SI5r, UB60r

SI warming: SI5t, UB60t, UB66r, SI2r

1. Indications

Taiyang Small Intestine meridian has cold energy from fire element. Heart and Small intestine have an internal-external relationship. Heart provides the fire nature of the blood with its Shaoyin fire energy while Small Intestine provides the water nature of the blood through its Taiyang cold energy. Yang organs work outside for Yin organ. Yin organs stay inside and provide a foundation to Yang organs. SI works for Heart and it distributes and moves the blood. Therefore, SI tonification can be used for blood deficiency as well as blood stagnation. SI meridian is connected to Small Intestine organ, so it can be used for SI disease and pain on SI meridian.

Headaches, vertigo, and insomnia due to blood deficiency can be treated with Small intestine tonification. Infertility due to blood deficiency or blood stagnation can be treated with SI tonification as well.

For bleeding disorder due to blood heat or blood stagnation, Taiyang cold energy of Small Intestine meridian can cool the blood heat, and Small intestine moves the blood stagnation.

Small intestine tonification also can be used for dryness of eyes, nose, mouth, and skin due to blood deficiency.

Urinary disorder due to Small intestine heat can be treated with Small intestine tonification or cooling formula when Taiyang Urinary Bladder heat is transferred from Taiyang Small intestine.

2. Case studies

- A 59-year-old, thin female suffered from a left shoulder pain. Abduction of left arm was possible only up to 90 degrees with difficulty. Such pain had begun since she had traumatized her left shoulder. Pain seemed to be due to trauma causing blood stasis. Pain location corresponded with Small Intestine meridian flow. Hand Taiyang Small Intestine tonification was used on the right side in order to break blood stagnation. Almost full abduction was achieved after a few treatments.

- A 29-year-old male had a pain all over the body after having a motorcycle accident. There was a slight heat sensation around pain location. It was considered to be trauma causing blood stasis. Hand Taiyang Small Intestine tonification was used. After 2 treatments, the pain disappeared.

- A 16-year-old male, 5'7" and 100lbs, suffered from strain on fifth metacarpal-phalangeal joint of right hand. Hand Taiyang Small Intestine tonification was used on the left side. The pain was alleviated to a certain extent after a few treatments.

- A 22-year-old female, 5'4" and 108lbs, had an amenorrhea for 3 months. She had a slightly red complexion. She seemed to be very alert and sensitive. She was worried a lot over trivial things and could not easily take a rest. She had fatigue, heat sensation rising from lower abdomen and spontaneous sweating. Her tongue was red and pulse was flooding, wiry, and slightly rapid. It was considered to be heat in the heart. Hand Taiyang Small Intestine meridian was chosen since the symptoms were closely related to blood. Hand Taiyang Small Intestine tonification and the sedation of HT8 were used. The treatment was very effective.

Foot Taiyang Urinary Bladder Meridian

UB tonification: UB67t, LI1t, SUB40r, ST36r

UB sedation: UB40t, ST36t, UB65r, UB41r

UB cooling: UB66t, SI2t, SI5r, UB60r

UB warming: SI5t, UB60t, UB66r, SI2r

1. Indications

Taiyang Urinary Bladder meridian has cold energy from the water element of the organ. Taiyang cold energy cools down fire. This is the coldest meridian in the body. Since Urinary Bladder meridian is connected to Urinary Bladder organ, it can be used for Urinary Bladder disease as well as pain along Urinary Bladder meridian.

Taiyang cold energy can treat any kind of heat symptoms. With Urinary Bladder tonification, redness of eyes due to Yin deficient fire can be treated since Urinary Bladder meridian starts on the inner canthus of eyes.

Pain on the area along the Urinary Bladder meridian can be treated with Taiyang Urinary Bladder tonification, such as neck stiffness, lower back pain, and occipital headaches. Especially the lower back pain caused by Kidney Yin deficiency can be treated with Urinary Bladder tonification.

Urinary Bladder meridian is connected with Urinary Bladder organ, so Urinary Bladder disease such as Urinary disorders, cystolithiasis, and urolithiasis can be treated with Urinary Bladder meridian.

Since Urinary Bladder's Taiyang cold energy can also tonify Yin, irregular menstruation caused by Kidney Yin deficiency can be treated with Urinary Bladder tonification.

2. Case studies

- A 27-year-old male, married for 3 months, suffered from a severe lower back pain. Pain had occurred a few days ago without an apparent reason. He had red eyes and fever all over the body. His pulse was rapid. Excessive sexual activity was considered to be the cause. Pain and heat sensation were reduced after a treatment of Urinary Bladder tonification, and gradually improved further with more treatments.

- A 64-year-old male, 5'6" and 100lbs, had high blood pressure and soreness in the lower back. He smoked a pack of cigarette a day. Foot Taiyang Urinary Bladder tonification was used since the pain location corresponded with Urinary Bladder meridian flow and also it clears heat.

55. A 38-year-old male, 5'8" and 145lbs, had suffered from stiff neck, which occurred after exposing to the rain for a long hour. He also complained of a chronic spinal

pain and occasional diarrhea. He had cold limbs. Foot Taiyang Urinary Bladder warming formula was used and Du 26 was added. Stiffness was alleviated and it completely disappeared after 3 treatments.

Hand Shaoyin Heart Meridian

HT tonification: LV1t, HT9t, KD10r, HT3r

HT sedation: KD10t, HT3t, SP3r, HT7r

HT cooling: KD10t, HT3t, HT8r, KD2r

HT warming: HT8t, KD2t, KD10r, HT3r

1. Indications

Shaoyin Heart meridian has monarch fire energy from fire element. Fire energy can warm up coldness. Heart meridian is connected with Heart organ. Therefore, it can be used for Heart disease. Also, Heart governs the "Shen", so it can be used for mental disorders.

Shaoyin monarch fire energy can treat coldness.

It also can be utilized for heart related diseases such as arrhythmia and angina.

It can treat mental disorder since Heart governs the spirit.

2. Case studies

- A 56-year-old female had deep and slow pulse. She had

a pain in the chest, palpitation, bodyaches, swelling, and profuse sweating. Such symptoms were considered to be Heart deficiency. The symptoms got improved after hand Shaoyin Heart tonification was applied.

57. A 27-year-old female suffered from insomnia and skin eruptions after having a serious mental anguish about 2 months ago. The eruption was spread around her lips and lower half of the face. There was a slight heat sensation on eruptions. She also had a forgetfulness and irritability. She was quick tempered and impatient. It was considered to be Heart excess. Foot Taiyang Urinary Bladder tonification and Hand Shaoyin Heart sedation were used and some improvements were observed.

• A 50-year-old female had a red face, hypertension, stifling sensation in the chest and sighed a lot. Her pulse was weak and rapid. The red face and irritability were considered to be heart deficient fire symptoms. Hand Shaoyin Heart tonification was used. With 3 treatments the red face and sighing were improved.

• A 35-year-old female was worried over every little thing. Recently she lost her husband and suffered from palpitation and irritability. Her pulse was intermittent. After Hand Shaoyin Heart tonification treatments, pulse was restored and she could easily fall asleep at night.

Foot Shaoyin Kidney Meridian

KD tonification: LU8t, KD7t, SP3r, KD3r

KD sedation: SP3t, KD3t, LV1r, KD1r

KD cooling: KD10t, HT3t, HT8r, KD2r

KD warming: HT8t, KD2t, KD10r, HT3r

1. Indications

Shaoyin Kidney meridian has Monarch fire energy of Shaoyin from Water element of the organ. It can warm up and nourish the body at the same time. Since Kidney is prone to deficiency, Kidney sedation is hardly ever used in the clinical situation. Kidney meridian is connected to Kidney organ, so Kidney tonification can be used for Kidney related diseases as well as Kidney deficiency.

Kidney deficient symptoms include tinnitus, low back pain, dysuria, lower abdominal cold pain, diarrhea, edema, weakness of the legs, irregular menstruation, and infertility.

2. Case studies

- A 25-year-old thin male suffered from lower back pain. He had a pale complexion. The pain was considered to be from excessive sexual activity. The pain was reduced after Foot Shaoyin Kidney tonification.

- A female suffered from a cold body and weakness in joints all over the body ever since having a second child. She also complained of recent problems such as irregular menses and cold hands. She was considered to be a cold constitution with Kidney deficiency. With 2-3 treatments on Foot Shaoyin Kidney tonification, her extremities had warmed up and other symptoms were improved.

- An 18-year-old female suffered from red spots on the skin. Originally there was only a slight irritation and itching when she put her hands in cold water, but from 2 years ago the red spots started to occur after exposing to the cold air. Recently it had spread over the face, neck and back region. The symptoms were more severe during autumn and winter season. Usually, skin diseases are caused by heat, bur in this case true yin and false yang with cold dryness were considered to cause the symptoms. Foot Shaoyin Kidney tonification was used and an improvement was observed.

Hand Shaoyang San Jiao Meridian

SJ tonification: GB41t, SJ3t, UB66r, SJ2r

SJ sedation: UB66t, SJ2t, ST36r, SJ10r

SJ cooling: UB66t, SJ2t, SI5r, SJ6r

SJ warming: SI5t, SJ6t, UB66r, 2r

1. Indications

Hand Shaoyang San Jiao meridian has fire energy. San Jiao is a functional organ, not an anatomical organ. Shaoyang ministerial fire is more active than monarch fire. The function of Shaoyang energy is warming, exciting and dispersing. It is very hot and dry, so Shaoyang San Jiao tonification can treat cold dampness. Also, it can be used for pain on San Jiao meridian.

Shaoyang ministerial fire disperses stagnation, raises Qi and excites the emotion. Therefore, it can be applied for depression.

The pain area on San Jiao meridian can be treated with Sanjiao tonification. The shoulder pain with cold dampness can get better with San Jiao tonification, while the shoulder pain with damp heat can be improved with Large Intestine tonification. For the shoulder pain with blood stagnation, Small intestine tonification can be applied.

Headaches caused by coldness, especially Jueyin vertex headaches, can be treated with Shaoyang San Jiao tonification.

Hair loss caused by cold dampness can be treated with San Jiao tonification, while hair loss from Kidney deficiency can be treated with Kidney tonification.

Shaoyang ministerial fire warms up, raises up, and brightens, so dimness of eyes from cold dampness and yang Qi deficiency can be treated with San Jiao tonification as well.

Leukorrhea caused by cold dampness can also be treated with San Jiao tonification.

2. Case studies

- A 50-year-old female lost her son by an accident and suffered from a mental shock. She complained of insomnia and pain in the chest and shoulder. Hand Shaoyang San Jiao tonification was used and she could sleep well afterward.

- A 30-year-old obese male complained of stiff neck after taking a shower with cold water. It was considered to be a cold attack. The symptom was alleviated after hand Shaoyang San Jiao tonification was applied and got completely cured after 3 treatments.

- A 37-year-old male had failed in business by his friend's betrayal. He had suffered from headaches, dull speech with stiff tongue, and insomnia ever since that incident. Shock from the betrayal seemed to be the cause of all problems. Hand Shaoyang San Jiao tonification was administered. After a few treatments, headaches were disappeared and he could speak and sleep better.

66. A 46-year-old female suffered from a left shoulder pain. She could not lift her left arm more than 45 degrees. Hand Shaoyang San Jiao tonification was used since the pain location corresponded with San Jiao meridian flow. There was a significant improvement after one treatment.

Foot Shaoyang Gall Bladder Meridian

GB tonification: UB66t, GB43t, LI1r, GB44r

GB sedation: LI1t, GB44t, SI5r, GB38r

GB cooling: UB66t, GB43t, SI5r, GB38r

GB warming: SI5t, GB38t, UB66r, GB43r

1. Indications

Shaoyang Gall Bladder meridian has fire energy from wood element. Shaoyang ministerial fire has warming and drying function, therefore used for cold dampness. Since Shaoyang Gall Bladder meridian is connected to Gall Bladder organ, it can be used for GB diseases as well as the pain on the Gall Bladder meridian. Although tonification is used more than sedation, the sedation formula is still used commonly in the treatment of Gall Bladder meridian.

Migraine, caused by Shaoyang fire, can be treated with Gall Bladder sedation.

Pain on the Gall Bladder meridian such as sciatica can be treated with GB meridian formulas. When there is cold dampness, GB tonification is better to use.

Shaoyang ministerial fire warms up, raises up, and brightens, so dimness of eyes due to cold dampness, Yang Qi deficiency, or GB deficiency can be treated with GB tonification.

Gall Bladder energy gives excitement and bravery. Therefore, GB tonification can be applied for mental and emotional disorder such as fear, melancholia, and depression, while GB sedation can be applied for anxiety and irritability.

Indigestion due to cold dampness can be treated with GB tonification.

Leukorrhea due to cold dampness can be treated with GB tonification.

Impotence, caused by Yang deficiency with cold dampness, can be treated with GB tonification.

Tinnitus, caused by Shaoyang excess, can be treated with GB sedation.

2. Case studies

- A 43-year-old female suffered from severe left abdominal pain. She also complained of dry mouth and throat, reduced appetite, indigestion, scanty dark urine, burning sensation in the anus, and migraine. She had a surgery for removal of gall stones 2 years ago. Her pulse was slightly rapid. Migraine was gone after 2 treatments of foot Shaoyang Gall Bladder sedation. Abdominal pain was also alleviated.

- A thin female in her late 40s, who is pharmacist, complained of chronic indigestion and abdominal distention. Her extremities were cold and pulse was very slow. There also was an occasional lower back pain due to cold excess. Indigestion and distention showed significant improvements with 3 treatments of foot Shaoyang Gall Bladder tonification. All the above symptoms were alleviated with additional treatments.

69. A 27-year-old female complained of dry mouth with bad breath. She had difficulty in ingesting foods and insomnia. She often woke up with unpleasant dreams. She easily sweated and always felt tired. She mentioned that she had an abortion for having a deformed

baby and lost her close friend by an accident. Both happened last year. It was considered to be constraint fire rising. Foot Shaoyang Gall Bladder sedation was used. Insomnia and other symptoms were gradually improved with additional treatments.

Hand Jueyin Pericardium meridian

PC tonification: LV1t, PC9t, KD10r, PC3r

PC sedation: KD10t, PC3t, SP3r, PC7r

PC cooling: KD10t, PC3t, HT8r, PC8r

PC warming: HT8t, PC8t, KD10r, PC3r

1. Indications

Jueyin Pericardium meridian has wind energy. Wind energy has converging and absorbing function. Pericardium is closely related with Heart and mind. It calms down the disturbed Shen(神) and improves the memory. Also, it can be used for pain on Pericardium meridian.

Pericardium tonification can be used for unconsciousness and dementia since it calms down the disturbed Shen.

Aphasia and Stuttering can also be treated with Pericardium tonification due to its ability to strengthening the Shen.

Pericardium tonification improves the memory and can be used for forgetfulness.

2. Case studies

- A 43-year-old male suffered from left shoulder pain, frequent coughing, and the itchy throat. Such symptoms had developed after gas poisoning 3 months ago. He became misty minded afterward. Hand Jueyin Pericardium tonification was used.

- A 50-year-old male suffered from strained pain in Biceps muscle after having a cold. The pain seemed most likely from the toxicity, from the latent heat remaining in the body. The pain location corresponded with Pericardium Meridian. Hand Jueyin Pericardium tonification was administered and the pain was subsided.

- A Patient had developed numbness in the middle finger from the location of PC9 and his chief complaint was difficult speech. Hand Jueyin Pericardium tonification was used. Numbness was disappeared and he could speak better.

Foot Jueyin Liver meridian

LV tonification: LV8t, KD10t, LV4r, LU8r

LV sedation: LU8t, LV8t, HT8r, LV2r

LV cooling: KD10t, LV8t, HT8r, LV2r

LV warming: HT8t, LV2t, KD10r, LV8r

1. Indications

Jueyin Liver meridian has wind energy from wood element. Liver Jueyin energy has characteristics such as sour taste, astringing, softening, and moistening. Liver stores the blood through the Jueyin energy and maintain the free flow of Qi with the help of Gall Bladder. Liver tonification can treat blood deficiency by strengthening the blood storing function of Liver. Liver Jueyin meridian is connected to Liver so Liver disease can also be treated with Liver meridian treatment.

Liver controls the tendons, so the weakness of the tendons and tiredness of four limbs can be treated with Liver tonification.

Liver related disease such as Liver cirrhosis can be treated with Liver meridian.

Headaches due to blood deficiency can also be treated with Liver tonification.

Liver opens into the eyes. Liver blood nourishes the eyes and Gall Bladder Shaoyang energy brightens the vision. Eye diseases like dryness of eyes and blurred vision caused by Liver blood deficiency can be treated with Liver tonification.

Liver channel curves around the external genitalia. Therefore, the external genital problem can be treated with Liver Channel.

2. Case studies

- A 37-year-old male suffered from swollen external genitalia. There was an occasional itching and white discharge came out. He had hypogastric pain and fatigue. Foot Jueyin Liver tonification was used and it was effective.

- A 30-year-old female complained of skin itching. The skin was very dry. IT would be irritated and easily get bruised if she scratched it. Such symptoms had begun 3 years ago when she was 3 months pregnant. She had cold body and she often experience static electricity during autumn and winter. Her pulse was weak and slightly rapid. It was considered to be yin deficiency because there was only itching without any eruptions and the itching was worse at night. Foot Jueyin Liver tonification was used to astringe and store body fluid.

- A 62-year-old male suffered from chronic hemorrhage and hemorrhoid. He was thin and pulse was weak. Among Points for foot Jueyin Liver tonification, only tonification of LV8 and sedation of LV4 were used. Fistula and bleeding symptoms were reduced by half after the treatment. With additional treatments, he got completely cured.

CHAPTER 4

CONCLUSION

The Korean Constitutional Acupuncture, Joseon acupuncture, and Sa Ahm acupuncture can be used not only for treating musculoskeletal problems but also for regulating hormones and immunity. While Joseon acupuncture technique is recommended to use only for the patients of over 50 years old with stubborn conditions such as degeneration of joints or spinal discs, KCA and Sa Ahm acupuncture can be used for anyone from infants to seniors.

That is why constitutional differentiation is the first step done in my clinic as soon as a patient walks in the clinic. You will also see more lasting treatment effect when you are on the right track in differentiating the constitution. Even when you select the points from Sa Ahm formulas, it is extremely beneficial to figure out the patient's constitution including the excess and deficiency of each element since both KCA and Sa Ahm acupuncture utilize 5 Shu points. The appearance of a patient tells you 60-70% information on his or her body type once you become more skilled and experienced, although it was emphasized in the first chapter that constitutional diagnosis should be made comprehensively based on all three of the appearances, the nature of the disposition, and the pathological symptoms. Therefore, it is crucial to pay attention to the physical image of patients including voice.

During the inspection of a patient, two dominant elements need to be found among wood, earth, metal, and water. This is the process to differentiate the constitutions based on 8 constitutional theory because in terms of practicing acupuncture, 8 constitutional differentiation works better than 4 constitutional theory to balance the elements more precisely.

There are tips to figure out the qualities of a dominant element. These are not absolute measurements, but it is at least much more tangible than pulse diagnosis and would help develop more objective standard of constitutional differentiation. Some tips might be overlapped with those described in the first chapter of this book. To improve the diagnostic success rate, comprehensive studies are required after understanding the qualities of each dominant element.

1. The Metal dominant qualities

- Shoulder: broad. Humerus head protrudes.
- Muscle Trapezius is well developed.
- Waste area is weak.
- Gluteus Medius muscle is not well developed.
- Strong voice. Good at singing. Tend to be talkative.
- Thin hairs.
- Upper portion of the head is well developed.
- Sharp and piercing eyes creating an intense and

aggressive look
- Due to the lack of bile production in the Gall bladder, it is harder for them to digest meat, fried food, or dairies.
- Cannot hold their liquor
- Tend to lose weight easily due to the difficulty in absorption of nutrition in the Small Intestine.

2. The Wood dominant qualities

- Shoulder: relatively narrow. Humerus head is relatively flat.
- Muscle Trapezius is not well developed.
- Waste area is well developed.
- Gluteus Medius muscle is well developed.
- Weak or raspy voice. Hard to sing high notes. Tend to be reserved.
- Mid to low portion of the face is well developed.
- It is easy for them to digest meat, fried food, or dairies. Tend to get gall stones easily. Over consumption of green leafy vegetable can cause Kidney stones for this type. Kidney stone analysis shows it.
- Tend to hold their liquor
- Tend to gain weight easily due to the well absorption of nutrition in the Small Intestine.

3. The Earth dominant qualities

- Chest area is well developed. (Broader and thicker)
- Tend to have smaller pelvis.
- Gluteus Maximus tends to be lifted and tighter.
- Tend to be short stature with smaller feet.

- Well defined and tighter calf muscle.
- Muscles are well developed in general.
- Their eyes also radiate a sharp and intense look.

4. The Water dominant qualities

- Chest area is not well developed. (Narrower and thinner)
- Tend to have bigger pelvis.
- Gluteus Maximus tends to be droopy and looser.
- Tend to be tall stature with bigger feet.
- Smooth and slimmer calf muscle.
- Muscles are not well developed in general.
- Tend to have enlarged prostate easily.

5. Examples (combined with Joseon acupuncture)

- Lumbar Radiculopathy

Male, 67 years old, Hispanic, 5'5", 205 lbs.

This patient came in for his low back pain. He is retired and has had back pain on and off for more than 10 years. His pain has gotten worse recently and he was diagnosed with Spinal stenosis with disc degeneration in the lumbar spine between L4 and L5. The pain also radiates down to the right leg and foot.

His medical history includes asthma, gallstone, high blood pressure, high cholesterol. His waste area and Gluteus Medius muscle is well developed.
His voice is raspy. Mid to low portion of his face is well

developed.

He has no problem in digesting meat, fried food, or dairies. He tends to gain weight easily, and his primary doctor recommended him to lose weight because he is obese. Based on above information, his first dominant element is wood.

He is on the shorter side as a man, and His skin has resilience. His Gluteus Maximus on the tighter side. Therefore, His second dominant element is Earth.

According to Sasang Constitutional Medicine theory this patient is Tai Yin body type, and the hyperactive state of Wood leads to a hypoactive state of Metal. Therefore, his weakest element is Metal.

On the perspective of Eight constitutional acupuncture, this patient belongs to Heat Tai Yin Constitution (AKA. Wood Yin body type), which is Tai Yin type with Shao Yang quality.
   The order of his organ strength is as below.

Liver > Heart > Spleen > Kidney >Lung
Gall Bladder > Small Intestine >Stomach> Urinary Bladder > Large Intestine

For the pain control, the points used are LI1t, UB67t, SI5r, and UB60r, with 0.20x15mm needles.

Since the disc degeneration in the lumbar spine was mainly between L4 and L5, Du3 and Extra15 next to Du3 were added with 0.35x60mm needles with gentle manipulation of rotating the needle backward and forward, evenly and continuously.

- Frozen shoulder

Female, 55 years old, Caucasian, 5'6", 133 lbs.

She came in for her left shoulder pain with limited range of motion. The abduction of her left shoulder was only 110 degrees. The pain had been getting worse and she was diagnosed with adhesive capsulitis. She used to be a flight attendant, and is currently a homemaker.
She has been taking digestive enzymes due to poor digestion. She is also lactose intolerant and sensitive to caffeine.
She states that she used to be very thin but recently gained some weight.
She is very talkative and her voice is clear.
Based on above information, her first dominant element is water, and her second dominate element is Metal.

According to Sasang Constitutional Medicine theory this patient is Shao Yin body type, and the hyperactive state of Water leads to a hypoactive state of Earth. Therefore, her weakest element is Earth.

On the perspective of Eight constitutional acupuncture, this patient belongs to Heat Shao Yin Constitution (AKA. Water Yang body type), which is Shao Yin type with Tai Yang quality

The order of her organ strength is as below.

Kidney > Lung > Liver >Heart > Spleen
Urinary Bladder > Large Intestine > Small Intestine > Gall Bladder > Stomach

For the pain control, the points used are SI5t, LI5t, UB66r, and LI2r, with 0.20x15mm needles.

In order to promote strong circulation in the left shoulder, LI16 (Jugu 巨骨), Extra point Jianzhong, and Ext23 (Jianqian 肩前) were added with 0.30x50mm needles with gentle manipulation of rotating the needle backward and forward, evenly and continuously.

· Hand tremors with cervicalgia

Female, 63 years old, Asian, 4'11", 90 lbs.

Her chief complaint is tremors in her both hands, and she also has other complaints like neck pain, back pain, and stiffness in the legs. The most pain is in her neck, diagnosed with disc degeneration between C7 and T1. The pain also radiates to the shoulders and arms.

She is very petite and both Gluteus Maximus and Medius are not well developed. She says she eats well, but still loses weight very easily. She has dry skin, very thin hair and could see her scalp through her hair all over.

Based on above information, her first dominant element is Metal.

She is short, and her muscles are relatively on the tighter side considering her age. Therefore, her second dominant element is Earth.

According to Sasang Constitutional Medicine theory this patient is Tai Yang body type, and the hyperactive state of Metal leads to a hypoactive state of Wood. Therefore, his weakest element is Wood.

On the perspective of Eight constitutional acupuncture, this patient belongs to Heat Tai Yang Constitution (Tai Yang type with Shao Yang quality), which is Metal Yang body type, Pulmotonia.

The order of her organ strength is as below

Lung > Spleen > Heart > Kidney > Liver
Large Intestine>Stomach >Small Intestine >Urinary Bladder
> Gall Bladder

For the balancing of her organ strength, the points used are LV8t, LV4r, KD10t, and LU8r, with 0.20x15mm needles. This is same as the Liver tonification formula in Sa Ahm acupuncture. Her condition of dry skin, thin hair, and tremors can be explained as symptoms due to blood deficiency and wind, based on Sa Ahm theory.

However, keep in mind that identifying the patient's constitution takes precedence over diagnosing based on the symptoms.

Since the disc degeneration mainly between C7 and T1, Du14 and GB20 were added with 0.25x40mm needles with gentle manipulation of rotating the needle backward and forward, evenly and continuously. The smaller gauge of needle is used considering her body size.

In all of the above cases, there were significant improvements in terms of the level of pain, the frequency of pain, the range of motion, and the tremors.

APPENDIX

As discussed in my other book <New Paradigms for Shang Han Lun>, Dr. Lee Jema concluded that Dr Zhang invented formulas for Shao Yin body type almost 100 percent. Therefore, it is recommended to prescribe Shang Han Lun formula actively for Shaoyins include Water Yin and Water Yang body type. However, Dr. Zhang barely obtained formulas for Tai Yin Body type, so the constitutional formulas of Dr. Lee need to be utilized more constructively for Taiyins including Wood Yin and Wood Yang body type. Here are the formulas of Dr. Lee Jema for all 4 constitutions.

Formulas of Sasang Constitutional Medicine

1. Formulas for Shao Yin body type

Exterior Syndrome

<u>Formulas for Exterior Excess Syndrome</u>

Chuan Xiong Gui Zhi Tang (川芎桂枝湯)   *Chuanxiong*
Rhizoma and Cinnamon Twig Decoction

Sheng Jiang 12, Gui Zhi 8, Ban Xia 8, Bai Shao 4, Bai Zhu 4, Chen Pi 4, Zhi Gan Cao 4

Huo   Xiang   Zheng   Qi   San   (藿香正氣散)
Agastache Powder to Rectify the Qi

Huo Xiang 6, Zi Su Ye 4, Cang Zhu 2, Bai Zhu 2, Ban Xia 2, Chen Pi 2, Qing Pi 2, Da Fu Pi 2, Gui Zhi 2, Gan Jiang 2, Yi Zhi Ren 2, Zhi Gan Cao 2

Ba   Wu   Jun   Zi   Tang   (八物君子湯)
Eight Noble Ingredients Decoction

Ren Shen 8, Huang Qi 4, Bai Zhu 4, Bai Shao 4, Dang Gui 4, Chuan Xiong 4, Chen Pi 4, Zhi Gan Cao 4, Sheng Jiang 4, Da Zao 3

Formulas for Exterior Deficiency Syndrome (Collapsed Yang in SCM)

Bu   Zhong   Yi   Qi   Tang(補中益氣湯)
Tonify the Middle and Augment the Qi Decoction

Ren Shen 12, Huang Qi 12, Zhi Gan Cao 4, Bai Zhu 4, Dang Gui 4, Chen Pi 4, Sheng Jiang 4, Da Zao 3, Huo Xiang 1.2-2, Zi Su Ye 1.2-2,

Sheng   Yang   Yi   Qi   Tang   (升陽益氣湯)
Raise the Yang and Augment the Qi Decoction

Ren Shen 8, Gui Zhi 8, Huang Qi 8, Bai Shao 8, Bai He Shou Wu 4, Rou Gui 4, Dang Gui 4, Zhi Gan Cao 4, Sheng Jiang 4, Da Zao 3

Interior Syndrome

Formulas for Tai Yin Syndrome

Gui   Zhi   Ban   Xia   Sheng   Jiang   Tang(桂枝半夏生薑湯)
Cinnamon Twig, Pinellia, and Fresh Ginger Decoction

Sheng Jiang 12, Gui Zhi 8, Ban Xia 8, Bai Shao 4, Bai Zhu 4, Chen Pi 4, Zhi Gan Cao 4

Chi Bai He Wu Guan Zhong Tang (赤白何烏寬中湯)　　　*Red*
and White Fo-Ti Root Decoction to Relieve the Middle

Bai He Shou Wu 4 Chi He Shou Wu 4 Gao Liang Jiang 4 Gan Jiang 4
Chen Pi 4 Qing

Bai He Shou Wu Li Zhong Tang (白何首烏理中湯)
Regulate the Middle Decoction with White Fo-Ti

Bai He shou Wu 8, bai zhu 8, Bai Shao 8, Gui Zhi 4, Gan Jiang 4,
Chen Pi 4, Zhi Gan Cao 4

Xiang Sha Yang Wei Tang (香砂養胃湯)　　　*Nourish the*
Stomach Decoction with Cyperus and Cardamon

Ren Shen 4, Bai Zhu 4, Bai Shao 4, Gan Cao 4, Ban Xia 4, Xiang Fu
4, Chen Pi 4, Gan Jiang 4, Shan Zha 4, Sha Ren 4, Bai Dou Kou 4,
Sheng Jiang 4, Da Zao 2

Huo Xiang Zheng Qi San (藿香正氣散)　　　*Agastache*
Powder to Rectify the Qi

Huo Xiang 6, Zi Su Ye 4, Cang Zhu 2, Bai Zhu 2, Ban Xia 2, Chen Pi
2, Qing Pi 2, Da Fu Pi 2, Gui Zhi 2, Gan Jiang 2, Yi Zhi Ren 2, Zhi Gan
Cao 2

Formulas for Shao Yin Syndrome

Guan Gui Fu Zi Li Zhong Tang (官桂附子理中湯)
Regulate the Middle Decoction with Cinnamon and Aconite

Ren Shen 12, Bai Zhu 8, Gan Jiang 8, Rou Gui 8, Bai Shao 4, Chen Pi
4, Zhi Gan Cao 4, Fu Zi 4-8

2. Formulas for Shao Yang body type

Exterior Syndrome

Formulas for Wind Attack Syndrome

Jing Fang Bai Du San (荊防敗毒散)   *Detoxify*
Pathogens Powder with Schizonepata and Siler

Qiang Huo 4 Du Huo 4 Chai Hu 4 Qian Hu 4 Jing Jie 4 Fang Feng 4
Chi Fu Ling 4 Sheng Di Huang 4 Di Gu Pi 4 Che Qian Zi 4

Jing Fang Dao Chi San (荊防導赤散)   *Guide Out the*
Red with Schizonepata and Siler Powder

Sheng Di Huang 12, Che Qian Zi 8, Xuan Shen 6, Gua Lou Ren 6,
Qian Hu 4, Qiang Huo 4, Du Huo 4, Jing Jie 4, Fang Feng 4

Jing Fang Xie Bai San (荊防瀉白散)   *Sedate the*
White with Schizonepata and Sileris Powder

Sheng Di Huang 12, Fu Ling 8, Ze Xie 8, Shi Gao 4, Zhi Mu 4, Qiang
Huo 4, Du Huo 4, Jing Jie 4, Fang Feng 4

Formulas for Collapsed Yin Syndrome (Mang Yin 亡陰)

Jing Fang Di Huang Tang (荊防地黃湯)   *Rehmannia*
with Schizonepata and Sileris Decoction

Shu Di Huang 8, Shan Zhu Yu 8, Fu Ling 8, Ze Xie 8, Che Qian Zi 4,
Qiang Huo 4, Du Huo 4, Jing Jie 4, Fang Feng 4

Hua Shi Ku Shen Tang (滑石苦蔘湯) *Talcum and Sophora Decoction*

Ze Xie 8, Fu Ling 8, Hua Shi 8, Ku Shen 8, Huang Lian 4, Huang Bai
4, Qiang Huo 4, Du Huo 4, Jing Jie 4, Fang Feng 4

Zhu Ling Che Qian Zi Tang (猪苓車前子湯) *Polyporus and Plantain Decoction*

Ze Xie 8, Fu Ling 8, Zhu Ling 6, Che Qian Zi 6, Zhi Mu 4, Shi Gao 4,

Qiang Huo 4, Du Huo 4, Jing Jie 4, Fang Feng 4,

Jing Fang Xie Bai San (荊防瀉白散)   *Sedate*
the White with Schizonepata and Sileris Powder

Sheng Di Huang 12, Fu Ling 8, Ze Xie 8, Shi Gao 4, Zhi Mu 4, Qiang Huo 4, Du Huo 4, Jing Jie 4, Fang Feng 4

Interior Syndrome

Formulas for Excess Yang Syndrome

Liang Ge San Huo Tang (凉膈散火)   *Cool the*
Diaphragm and Disperse the Fire Decoction

Sheng Di Huang 8 Ren Dong Teng 8 Lian Qiao 8 Zhi Zi 4 Bo He 4 Zhi Mu 4 Shi Gao 4 Fang Feng 4 Jing Jie 4

Ren   Dong   Teng   Di   Gu   Pi   Tang   (忍冬藤地骨皮湯)
Honeysuckle Stem and Lycium Bark Decoction

Ren Dong Teng 16, Shan Zhu Yu 8, Di Gu Pi 8, Huang Lian 8, Huang Bai 8, Xuan Shen 4, Ku Shen 4, Sheng Di Huang 4, Zhi Mu 4, Zhi Zi 4, Gou Qi Zi 4, Fu Pen Zi 4, Jing Jie 4, Fang Feng 4, Jin Yin Hua 4

Di Huang Bai Hu Tang (地黃白虎湯)   *White Tiger*
with Rehmannia Decoction

Shi Gao 20-40, Sheng Di Huang 16, Zhi Mu 8, Fang Feng 4, Du Huo 4

Formulas for Deficient Yin Syndrome

Shu   Di   Huang   Ku   Shen   Tang   (熟地黃苦蔘湯)
Rehmannia with Pubescent Angelica Decoction

Shu Di Huang 16, Shan Zhu Yu 8, Fu Ling 6, Ze Xie 6, Huang Bai 4, Ku Shen 4, Zhi Mu 4

Du　　　Huo　　　Di　　　Huang　　　Tang　　　(獨活地黃湯)
Rehmannia with Pubescent Angelica Decoction

Shu Di Huang 16, Shan Zhu Yu 8, Fu Ling 6, Ze Xie 6, Mu Dan Pi 4, Fang Feng 4, Du Huo 4

Shi　　　Er　　　Wei　　　Di　　　Huang　　　Tang　　　(十二味地黃湯)
Twelve Ingredients with Rehmannia Decoction

Shu Di Huang 16, Shan Zhu Yu 8, Fu Ling 6, Ze Xie 6, Mu Dan Pi 4, Di Gu Pi 4, Xuan Shen 4, Gou Qi Zi 4, Fu Pen Zi 4, Che Qian Zi 4, Jing Jie 4, Fang Feng 4

3. Formulas for Tai Yin body type

Exterior Syndrome

The Formulas for Exterior Cold

Ma　　　Huang　　　Fa　　　Biao　　　Tang　　　(麻黃發表湯)
Ephedra Decoction to Release Exterior

Jie Geng 12, Ma Huang 6, Mai Men Dong 4, Huang Qin 4, Xing Ren 4

Han　　　Duo　　　Re　　　Shao　　　Tang　　　(寒多熱少湯)
Greater Cold and Lesser Heat Decoction

Yi Yi Ren 12, Gan Li 12 (dried chest nut), Lai fu zi 8, Huang Qin 4, Mai Men Dong 4, Xing Ren 4, Jie Geng 4, Ma Huang 4

The Formulas for Cold Syndrome in the epigastrium

*Tai Yin Tiao Wei Tang*太陰調胃湯   *Decoction*
for Taiyins to Regulate the Stomach

Yi Yi Ren 12, Gan Li 12, Lai Fu Zi 8, Wu Wei Zi 4, Mai Men Dong 4, Shi Chang Pu 4, Jie Geng 4, Ma Huang 4

Tiao   *Wei*   *Cheng*   *Qing*   *Tang*(調胃升清湯)
Regulate the Stomach and Raise the Clear Decoction

Yi Yi Ren 12, Gan Li 12, Lai Fu Zi 6, Ma Huang 4, Jie Geng 4, Mai Men Dong 4, Wu Wei Zi 4, Shi Chang Pu 4, Yuan Zhi 4, Tian Men Dong 4, Suan Zao Ren 4, Long Yan Rou 4

Interior Syndrome

The Formulas for Dry Heat Syndrome

Ge   *Gen*   *Jie*   *Ji*   *Tang*   (葛根解肌湯)
Release the Muscle Layer Decoction with Kudzu

Ge Gen 12, Huang Qin 6, Gao Ben 6, Jie Geng 4, Sheng Ma 4, Bai Zhi 4

Re   *Duo*   *Han*   *Shao*   *Tang*   (熱多寒少湯)
Greater Heat and Lesser Cold Decoction

Ge Gen 16, Huang Qin 8, Gao Ben 8, Lai Fu Zi 4, Jie Geng 4, Sheng Ma 4, Bai Zhi 4

The Formuals for Yin Blood Exhaustion Syndrome

Lu   *Rong*   *Da*   *Bu*   *Tang*   (鹿茸大補湯)
Deer Antler Decoction for Great Tonification

Lu Rong 8-16, Mai Men Dong 6, Yi Yi Ren 6, Shan Yao 4, Tian Men Dong 4, Wu Wei Zi 4, Xing Ren 4, Ma Huang 4

Gong   Chen   He   Yuan   Dan   (拱辰黑元丹)
Modified Gong Chen Dan for Black Vitality

Lu Rong 16-24, Shan Yao 16, Tian Men Dong 16, Qi Cao 4-8

4. Formulas for Tai Yang body type

Exterior Syndrome

Formula for Jieyi (解㑊)

Wu   Jia   Pi   Zhuang   Ji   Tang   (五加皮壯脊湯)
Strengthen the Spine Decoction with Acanthopanax

Wu Jia Pi 16 Mu Gua 8 Qing Song Jie 8 Pu Tao Gen 4 Lu Gen 4 Ying Tao Rou 4 Qiao Mai Mi 4

Interior Syndrome

Formula for Yege(噎膈) or Fanwei(反胃)

Mi Hou Teng Zhi Chang Tang (獼猴籐植腸湯)   *Plant*
the Intestine Decoction with Actinidia

Mi Hou Tao 16, Mu Gua 8, Pu Tao Gen 8, Lu Gen 4, Ying Tao Rou 4, Wu Jia Pi 4, Song Hua 4, Chu Tou Tang(bran) 4

BIBLIOGRAPHY

Dr. Song Il-Byung, <An introduction to Sasang Constitutional Medicine> Seoul: Jipmoondang International, 2005

Lee Dongwoong, <The differentiation of 8 body types>, The association of Sasang constitution, 2001 (Korean Version)

Jeon Geumseon, Yoon Sijin, <Seokho Acupuncture Technique>, Shinheung Med Science

Kim Jongyeol and Duong Duc Pham, <Sasang Constitutional Medicine as a Holistic Tailored Medicine>

Sasang Constitutional Medicine, published by Jip Moon Dang (Korean Version)

Dr. Kuon Dowon, <Eight Constitutional Medicine : An overview>, Institute for Modern Korean Studies, 2003

Lee Gangjae, <The practice of Eight Constitutional Medicine>, Haeng Lim Seo Won 2009 (Korean version)

CMC research group, <The heavenly regimen>, Korea Medical, 2004 (Korean version)

Hiromichi Yasui, <Medical History in Japan>, The Journal of Kampo, Japan Institute of TCM Research, 2007

Lee Junghuan and Jung Changhyun, <Yakucho of Todo Yoshimasu>, Chung Hong, 2006 (Korean version)

Yumoto Kyushin, <Japanese-Chinese Medicine (Kokan Igaku)(Huang Han Yi Xue)>, Gye Chuk Moon Hwa Sa, 2015 (Korean version)

Yeom Taehwan, <The treatment with constitutional acupuncture>, WitGonni Company, 2007 (Korean version)

Cheng Xinnong, <Chinese Acupuncture and Moxibustion (revised edition)>, Foreign Languages Press, Beijing

Geum Oh Kim Hong Kyung, <An Invitation to Eastern Meidicine>, Shin Nong Baek Cho, 1990 (Korean Version)

Maoshing Ni, <The yellow emperor's classic of Medicine, Shambhala, Boston and London, 1995, p245

Kim Hong Kyung, <Revolution of Oriental Medicine>, Shin Nong Bon Cho press, Seoul, 1994, translated by Hugh Kim

www.musculoskeletalkey.com

Peter Baldry, <Superficial versus Deep Dry Needling>, , Aupuncture in Medicine 2002

www.unesco.org

Melanie Plenda, <Dry needling gives you that 'twitch response'>, The Union Leader, August 27, 2017
https://www.snhhealth.org/in-the-news/dry-needling-gives-you-that-twitch-response

Jun-Su Jang, Young-Su Kim, Boncho Ku, and Jong Yeol Kim,<Recent Progress in Voice-Based Sasang Constitutional Medicine: Improving Stability of Diagnosis>

Eunsu Jang, Jong Yeol Kim, Haejung Lee, Honggie Kim, Younghwa Baek, and Siwoo Lee,<A Study on the Reliability of Sasang Constitutional Body Trunk Measurement

http://www.hindawi.com/journals

Evidence-Based Complementary and Alternative Medicine
Volume 2013 (2013), Article ID 920384, 7 pages
http://dx.doi.org/10.1155/2013/920384

Evidence-Based Complementary and Alternative Medicine
Volume 2013 (2013), Article ID 920384, 7 pages
http://dx.doi.org/10.1155/2013/920384

Evidence-Based Complementary and Alternative Medicine

Volume 2012 (2012), Article ID 604842, 8 pages

http://dx.doi.org/10.1155/2012/604842

https://content.byui.edu/file/a236934c-3c60-4fe9-90aa-d343b3e3a640/1/
module10/readings/divisions_nerve_system.html#:~:text=DIVISIONS
%20OF%20THE%20AUTONOMIC%20NERVOUS%20SYSTEM
%20SYMPATHETIC%20DIVISION,the%20ventral%20root%20and%20enter
%20a%20spinal%20nerve.

A Modern Clinical Approach of the Traditional Korean Saam Acupuncture (hindawi.com) Scientific Evidence for Korean Medicine and Its Integrative Medical Research Volume 2015 Article ID 703439 | https://doi.org/10.1155/2015/703439 Manyong Park and Sungchul Kim

ACKNOWLEDGEMENT

First of all, I would like to convey my gratitude to the senior Traditional Asian Medicine practitioners who have built theoretical foundation of herbology and formula writing and have translated and interpreted the old text into the modern version, and to Korean Medicine doctors who compiled materials and shared their clinical studies for improvement of traditional Asian Medicine. I would also like to thank my husband and all my families for their unconditional love, support, and trust.

---

[1] The theory of 'internal energy, external shape (氣裏形表)' is from Dr. Heo Jun's 'Dongui Bogam (東醫寶鑑)'.
Dongui Bogam is traditional Korean Medicine book compiled by Dr. Heo and is on UNESCO's Memory of the World Programme as of July 2009.
[2] Dr. Kang Joobong, <The dynamics of Shang Han Lun>, published by IOMRI

[3] Known in English as 'The treatise on Cold injury'. Is a Chinese medical treatise that was compiled by Dr. Zhang ZhongJing sometime before the year 220. Is amongst the oldest complete clinical textbooks in the world.

[4] Dr. Song Il-Byung, <Basic Principles of SaSang Medicine>

[5] Kim Jongyeol and Duong Duc Pham, <Sasang Constitutional Medicine as a Holistic Tailored Medicine>

[6] Yeom Taehwan, <The treatment with constitutional acupuncture>, WitGonni Company,2007 (Korean version)

[7] Cheng Xinnong, <Chinese Acupuncture and Moxibustion (revised edition)>, Foreign Languages Press, Beijing, p7

[8] The effects of acupuncture needling on connective tissue, Helene M. Langevin, www.musculoskeletalkey.com

[9] <Superficial versus Deep Dry Needling>,Peter Baldry, Aupuncture in Medicine 2002; 20(2-3): 78-81

[10] www.unesco.org

[11] DIVISIONS OF THE AUTONOMIC NERVOUS SYSTEM
https://content.byui.edu/file/a236934c-3c60-4fe9-90aa-d343b3e3a640/1/module10/
readings/divisions_nerve_system.html#:~:text=DIVISIONS%20OF%20THE%20AUTONOMIC
%20NERVOUS%20SYSTEM%20SYMPATHETIC%20DIVISION,the%20ventral%20root%20and
%20enter%20a%20spinal%20nerve.

[12] <Dry needling gives you that 'twitch response'>, By Melanie Plenda,
The Union Leader, August 27, 2017
https://www.snhhealth.org/in-the-news/dry-needling-gives-you-that-twitch-response

[13] Y. O. Jung, D. H. Lee, and S. W. Ahn, "A research for tradition and identity of Saam acupuncture method," *Korean Journal of Acupuncture*, vol. 29, no. 4, pp. 537–553, 2012.

[14] A Modern Clinical Approach of the Traditional Korean Saam Acupuncture (hindawi.com) Scientific Evidence for Korean Medicine and Its Integrative Medical Research Volume 2015 Article ID 703439 | https://doi.org/10.1155/2015/703439 Manyong Park and Sungchul Kim

[15] A Modern Clinical Approach of the Traditional Korean Saam Acupuncture (hindawi.com) Scientific Evidence for Korean Medicine and Its Integrative Medical Research Volume 2015 Article ID 703439 | https://doi.org/10.1155/2015/703439 Manyong Park and Sungchul Kim

[16] J. W. Lee, The Secret of Sa-Ahm's Acupuncture Based on Yinyang and Five Elements, vol. 1, Institute for Studying Five Element Acupuncture, Busan, Republic of Korea, 1958.

[17] D. P. Kim, "Sa-Ahm's five element acupuncture and its usages," the Journals of the Korean Oriental Medical Society, pp. 122–123, 1972.

[18] S. H. Cho, The Systematic Research of Saam Acupuncture, Seongbo, 2001

[19] D. W. Kwon, "Constitutional acupuncture," The International Journal of Acupuncture and Moxibustion, pp. 149–167, 1965.

[20] H. K. Kim, Revolutionary Review of Oriental Medicine, Sinlong-Bonche, Seoul, Republic of Korea, 2001.

[21] Maoshing Ni, The yellow emperor's classic of Medicine, Shambhala, Boston and London, 1995, p245

[22] Four needle technique: Saam   www.taijiclub.live